NCTRC®

Exam Practice Questions

AF834553

Mometrix
TEST PREPARATION

Dear Future Exam Success Story

First of all, **THANK YOU** for purchasing Mometrix study materials!

Second, congratulations! You are one of the few determined test-takers who are committed to doing whatever it takes to excel on your exam. **You have come to the right place.** We developed these practice tests with one goal in mind: to deliver you the best possible approximation of the questions you will see on test day.

Standardized testing is one of the biggest obstacles on your road to success, which only increases the importance of doing well in the high-pressure, high-stakes environment of test day. Your results on this test could have a significant impact on your future, and these practice tests will give you the repetitions you need to build your familiarity and confidence with the test content and format to help you achieve your full potential on test day.

Your success is our success

We would love to hear from you! If you would like to share the story of your exam success or if you have any questions or comments in regard to our products, please contact us at **800-673-8175** or **support@mometrix.com**.

Thanks again for your business and we wish you continued success!

Sincerely,
The Mometrix Test Preparation Team

Written and edited by the Mometrix Exam Secrets Test Prep Team
Printed in the United States of America

TABLE OF CONTENTS

Practice Test #1

1. According to Piaget's and similar theories of cognitive development, when can most people typically think abstractly enough to perform mental operations without using concrete objects?

a. Right from infancy
b. In early adulthood
c. Pre-teens to teens
d. Middle adulthood

2. According to Maslow, the highest level on the hierarchy of needs which people strive to achieve is:

a. safety.
b. love and belonging.
c. esteem.
d. self-actualization.

3. The brain of a newborn infant weighs around __ of the weight of an adult's brain.

a. 50%
b. 25%
c. 10%
d. 75%

4. Psychologist Erik Erikson developed the theory that throughout a person's life, they pass through 8 different psychosocial stages. The stage at which a child begins to express his independence is:

a. stage 1 – trust vs. mistrust.
b. stage 2 – autonomy vs. shame and doubt.
c. stage 3 – initiative vs. guilt.
d. stage 4 – industry vs. inferiority.

5. According to Erikson, during what period of life do people most often reflect on what they have/have not accomplished and feel an overall sense of either satisfaction or regret?

a. Adolescence
b. Young adulthood
c. Middle adulthood
d. Mature adulthood

6. Among the following, who would be most likely to attribute human behavior to a process of learning through exposure to environmental stimuli and the environmental results of one's responses?

a. B. F. Skinner
b. Sigmund Freud
c. Howard Gardner
d. Abraham Maslow

7. One's belief in his/her competence to achieve a goal was specifically defined as _____ by _____.

a. actualizing tendency; Carl Rogers
b. self-efficacy; Albert Bandura
c. self-actualization; Abraham Maslow
d. industry; Erik Erikson

8. Whose work has most contributed to the person-centered model of health and human services?

a. Lev Vygotsky
b. Erik Erikson
c. Carl Rogers
d. Kraus & Shank

9. Which model of health and human services is most likely to be followed with developmentally disabled populations?

a. The educational model
b. Psychosocial rehabilitation
c. The recovery model
d. The community model

10. The International Classification of Functioning (ICF) classifies

a. health, not disability.
b. health and disability.
c. disability, not health.
d. disability and functioning.

11. The WHO's ICF (International Classification of Functioning) can be used in providing TR and other services. Which of the following is an example of its use at the institutional level?

a. Communication with other practitioners/agencies
b. Needs assessments for limitations in participation
c. Environmental assessments for universal design
d. Planning and developing the needed services

12. Which of the following is NOT true regarding US Census results from 2020?

a. The state with the highest diversity index is California
b. The largest ethnic group of California is Hispanic/Latino
c. The largest ethnic group of the District of Columbia is Black/African American
d. Hispanics were the largest USA minority group

13. In order to become a Recreational Therapist, a person must first:

a. complete a certification course offered at many community and technical colleges.
b. obtain an Associate's Degree in a related field.
c. obtain a Bachelor's Degree in Recreational Therapy or a related field.
d. there are no formal education requirements to become a Recreational Therapist.

14. What is the definition of cultural encounter?

a. A negative interaction between a healthcare provider and someone who is of a different cultural background
b. Encouraging medical professionals to interact with those of a different cultural background from their own
c. A coordinated effort between two cultural groups to gather and work through their differences
d. The egocentric behaviors of a set of individuals who are intolerant of those from a different culture

15. Among four levels of cultural competency in RTs, which one is considered the highest?

a. Unconsciously competent
b. Consciously incompetent
c. Unconsciously incompetent
d. Consciously competent

16. In TR groups, which of the following would most reflect the systems theory concept of homeostasis?

a. How group members share or omit and process information
b. The rules that a group has developed regulating its behavior
c. If feedback in a group provokes conflict and system changes
d. The interdependence of members creating the group whole

17. If a patient shows cognitive difficulties with comprehension, following directions, remembering, reading, writing, and executive function, which statement is most accurate about a diagnosis?

a. Neuropsychological testing is necessary for differential diagnosis
b. These symptoms are all clearly related to an intellectual disability
c. Some aphasia or other language disorder is the most likely cause
d. The symptoms described are typically associated with dementia

18. An injury at which level of the spinal cord may allow the patient to operate a motorized wheelchair on their own?

a. C4
b. C5
c. C3
d. C2

19. Parents of a child with cerebral palsy who is now wheelchair-bound express their concerns about his ability to go to school. The recreational therapist should advise them that:

a. there are laws in place to ensure he has equal access to an education or special education despite his disabilities.
b. they will need to hire private tutors for him to be educated at home.
c. most children with cerebral palsy stop going to school once they are in a wheelchair.
d. there are inpatient facilities similar to boarding schools where he will have to go to earn a full education.

20. TR activities that focus on range of motion (ROM) are especially important for patients with:

a. spina bifida
b. muscular dystrophy
c. cerebral palsy
d. multiple sclerosis

21. For a patient who has had a stroke to the left hemisphere of the brain, which is a better TR practice?

a. To do more leisure education than reality orientation
b. To keep any distractions out of the TR environment
c. To use more verbal directions instead of gestures
d. To use more physical gestures instead of words

22. Of the following, which is categorized as a metabolic disorder?

a. Type 1 Diabetes mellitus
b. Phenylketonuria (PKU)
c. Cushing syndrome
d. Hyperthyroidism

23. How can infectious diseases be transmitted to humans?

a. Direct or indirect contact, contaminated food, or insect bites
b. They can be transmitted by direct contact, but not indirectly
c. Insect bites can transmit these, but not food contaminations
d. From contaminated food or insect bites but not from contact

24. If someone has a hearing loss caused only by otitis media, the type of hearing loss is:

a. conductive.
b. sensorineural.
c. mixed hearing loss.
d. impossible to identify.

25. When an individual's eyes do not focus together on the same point, what is this called?

a. Strabismus
b. Nystagmus
c. Presbyopia
d. Retinopathy

26. The diagnosis of obsessive-compulsive disorder (OCD) refers to which of these?

a. Obsessive thoughts and compulsive behaviors
b. Obsessive behaviors and compulsive thoughts
c. Obsessive rituals caused by compulsive fixations
d. Obsessive and compulsive thought and behavior

27. Which of the following is a common sign of drug abuse, but not necessarily of drug addiction?

a. Needing more of a drug to get the same effects as before
b. Getting into trouble with the law because of the drug use
c. Needing drugs to relieve or prevent withdrawal symptoms
d. Having lost control over how much or how often one uses

28. Of the following, which would best fit the legal requirement of Least Restrictive Environment (LRE)?

a. Children with disabilities are educated in regular classes using needed supports / services
b. Children with disabilities are educated in special classes that eliminate regular restrictions
c. Children with disabilities are educated in separate schools to eliminate regular restrictions
d. Children with disabilities are educated in regular classes with no restrictive added services

29. The federal Access Board enforces the Architectural Barriers Act (ABA) of 1968. This Board was established under which law?

a. Title III of the NCLB (2001) legislation
b. Title I of the NCLB's (2001) legislation
c. Section 502 of the Rehabilitation Act
d. Section 504 of the Rehabilitation Act

30. Which of the following is an example of a societal stereotype?

a. These are all actually examples of societal stereotypes
b. Believing all African-Americans are athletically superior
c. Believing all Asian people are naturally more intelligent
d. Believing all Asian individuals are always terrible drivers

31. Regardless of when each was first enacted, which of the following laws has had a *partial* update the most recently?

a. The Americans with Disabilities Act
b. Individuals with Disabilities Education Act
c. The Older Americans Act (OAA)
d. (A) and (B) had updates the same year

32. Currently there is legislation regulating TR/RT or physical and occupational therapy in

a. a number of states in the USA.
b. only the Federal government.
c. none of the states in the USA.
d. all of the states in the USA.

33. Ancient Greek philosopher Aristotle defined three levels of leisure. Which of these is NOT one?

a. The level of contemplation
b. The level of perceived freedom
c. The level of recreation
d. The level of amusement

34. According to many experts, which of the following is most often defined as not only enjoyable but also having morally acceptable and socially redeeming values?

a. Recreation
b. Leisure
c. Play
d. All

35. Relative to leisure across the life span, what is most accurate about "Core" vs. "Balance" activities?

a. Balance leisure activities give more variety
b. Core leisure activities change through life
c. Balance leisure activities usually cost less
d. Core leisure activities are less accessible

36. The literature from leisure research has established which of these?

a. People pursue more stability than novelty in their leisure experiences
b. People pursue more novelty than stability in their leisure experiences
c. People seek equal amounts of stability and novelty in leisure activities
d. People seek novelty in leisure when young and stability at older ages

37. Which concept of TR/RT places the most emphasis on addressing all of an individual's needs?

a. TR/RT as recreative experience
b. Special or adaptive recreation
c. The holistic approach to TR/RT
d. TR/RT as a treatment modality

38. Which NCTRC specialty certification area of practice can encompass populations from all the others?

a. Physical Medicine/Rehabilitation
b. Developmental Disabilities
c. Community Inclusion
d. Behavioral Health

39. Which of the following models of TR/RT LEAST follows a continuum of increasing independence for the participant?

a. The Treatment models
b. The Leisure Ability model
c. The Long-Term Care model
d. The Activity Therapy model

40. In the practice settings of group homes and prisons, which TR/RT model is most likely?

a. The Medical/Clinical model
b. The Milieu Therapy model
c. The Long-Term Care model
d. Education/Training model

41. The RT gathers culturally appropriate baseline data on patient/client strengths and weaknesses in physical, cognitive, emotional, behavioral, social, and leisure functioning. This is an example of which of the ATRA standards of practice?

a. Treatment planning
b. Ethical conduct
c. Assessment
d. Discharge

42. RTs are responsible for seeing that clients receive equal services regardless of financial status, social status, disability, disease, race, color, creed, gender, age, or sexual orientation. Which principle in the ATRA Code of Ethics reflects this?

a. Fidelity
b. Justice
c. Veracity
d. Autonomy

43. Which principle of the ATRA Code of Ethics for RT personnel stipulates that they protect the people they serve from harm?

a. Principle 5, Fidelity
b. Principle 10, Compliance with Laws and Regulations
c. Principle 2, Nonmaleficence
d. Principle 6, Veracity

44. If, for fear of discouraging the client, the recreational therapist omitted a little information about the client's prognosis in RT, this would violate which principle of the ATRA Code of Ethics?

a. None
b. Fidelity
c. Veracity
d. Justice

45. When assessing a client/patient, in which domain would the person's level of engagement belong?

a. Psychosocial
b. Affective
c. Cognitive
d. Physical

46. By observing a person's bodily gestures, facial expressions, and estimating the person's relative level of self-esteem, which domain of behavior can the RT best assess?

a. Psychosocial
b. Affective
c. Cognitive
d. Physical

47. Which assessment tool is used by Recreational Therapists in a short-term, psychiatric setting?

a. State Technical Institute Assessment Process (STIAP)
b. Leisure Barriers Inventories (LBI)
c. Minimum Data Set (MDS)
d. Comprehensive Evaluation in Recreational Therapy (CERT)

48. In order to place a patient into an appropriate therapeutic recreation program, the Recreation Therapist must perform an accurate and complete:

a. comprehensive assessment.
b. set of vital signs.
c. review of demographic information.
d. physical exam.

49. All of the following elements are part of the affective assessment EXCEPT for:

a. attitude toward self.
b. expression.
c. problem solving skills.
d. nonverbal communication cues.

50. Which assessment tool enables Recreation Therapists to measure someone's current level of leisure functioning?

a. Leisure Scope
b. Functional Assessment of Characteristic for TR (FACTR)
c. Life Satisfaction Scale (LSS)
d. Leisure Diagnostic Battery (LDB)

51. Which portion of the assessment performed by the Recreation Therapist involves evaluation of motor skills and functioning?

a. Sensory assessment
b. Physical assessment
c. Functional skills assessment
d. Social assessment

52. The assessment tool used by Recreation Therapists to evaluate how a patient views free time is the:

a. Leisure Activity Blank (LAB).
b. WHODAS.
c. Free Time Boredom Assessment.
d. Idyll Arbor Leisure Battery.

53. What is most accurate about assessment practices by RTs and other therapeutic fields?

a. About half of RTs use commercial standardized tests like CERT, FOX, REDS, LCM, LDB, or Leisurescope
b. More than half of physical therapists, like RTs, do not employ commercial standardized assessments
c. Some research finds mental health professionals monitor progress using only standardized measures
d. TR is unique among therapeutic fields in its practitioners' lack of using available standardized testing

54. Currently, the majority of practicing RTs are more likely to use which of these in assessment?

a. Neither clinical evaluation nor clinical judgment
b. Clinical evaluation and judgment in combination
c. Clinical evaluation rather than clinical judgment
d. Clinical judgment rather than clinical evaluation

55. Which part of the Leisure Assessment Inventory or LAI (Hawkins et al, 2002) helps the RT to determine how a client is limited from participating in certain leisure activities?

a. The Leisure Constraints Index (L-CON)
b. The Leisure Activity Participation Index (LAP)
c. The Leisure Preference Index (L-PREF)
d. The Leisure Interest Index (L-INT)

56. If an assessment instrument is valid, what does this mean?

a. It produces stable results when reused over time
b. It means the test will accomplish both (A) and (D)
c. It will consistently produce the same results
d. It measures what it means and claims to measure

57. Whether a test represents everything in the construct or behavior being measured is called:

a. Content validity
b. Construct validity
c. Convergent validity
d. Discriminant validity

58. Test authors want to validate their updated new version of an instrument. They give the old version to one group of students, and give the new version to another group of students at the same time. What kind of validity are they trying to establish?

a. Predictive validity
b. Concurrent validity
c. Construct validity
d. Content validity

59. Which of the following type of reliability is determined by computing a correlation coefficient?

a. Test-retest reliability
b. All these types of reliability
c. Equivalent forms reliability
d. Split-half reliability

60. An error of measurement that makes a test instrument less valid is what kind of error?

a. A constant error makes a test instrument less valid
b. A random error makes a test instrument less valid
c. Neither of these make a test instrument less valid
d. Either a constant or random error makes a test instrument less valid

61. Which of the following types of test reliability can be established with only one test administration?

a. Alternate-forms reliability
b. Test-retest reliability
c. All these types can
d. Split-half reliability

62. If the RT wants to determine which activities a client can participate in and gives a Leisure Interests assessment that reveals the client has a strong interest in a particular activity that s/he is permanently unable physically to participate in, this relates to which criterion for selecting the assessment?

a. Availability
b. Validity
c. Purpose
d. Reliability

63. In implementing assessment for TR/RT, which choice gives some of the steps in the correct order?

a. Reviewing the test protocol; analyzing the results; interpreting the results; documenting
b. Documenting; interpreting the results; analyzing the results; reviewing the test protocol
c. Analyzing the results; reviewing the test protocol; documenting; interpreting the results
d. Interpreting the results; reviewing the test protocol; documenting; analyzing the results

64. Which type of interview is most likely to include "Yes/No" questions?

a. Structured
b. Unstructured
c. Semi-structured
d. All are equally likely

65. When assessing whether a patient can read or is legally blind, whether the patient's hearing is within normal limits, and whether the patient is tactile-defensive, which functional domain is being assessed?

a. Cognitive
b. Sensory
c. Physical
d. Social

66. Assessment of physical, mental, emotional, behavioral, or social constraints to leisure activity relates most to assessment of:

a. leisure skills.
b. leisure values.
c. leisure barriers.
d. leisure interests.

67. The World Health Organization Disability Assessment Schedule (WHODAS 2.0) is used to measure which of the following?

a. The mental impact of disability
b. The level of health and disability within an individual
c. The risk factors for complications of disability
d. The origin of an individual's disability

68. For a patient with loss of sensation secondary to diabetes, which of the following demonstrates that the RT anticipates is a contraindication based on the patient's diagnosis?

a. Not allowing the patient to engage in physical exercise to prevent fatigue
b. Not allowing the patient to sit for long times without a release of pressure
c. Not allowing the patient to eat any food before or after physical activities
d. Not allowing the patient to engage in activities if blood sugar tests normal

69. Which of the following should the RT consider when working with patients who take seizure medications?

a. The patient may have trouble following directions
b. The patient may have any/all of these side-effects
c. The patient may be dizzy and lacking coordination
d. The patient may be short of breath and may faint

70. What is accurate about the Intake Assessment Report in the field of TR/RT?

a. Only a certain approved professional can generate the intake assessment report
b. In community settings, a doctor's prescription takes precedence over this report
c. It is unlikely to inform the RT's identifying suitable interview topics and questions
d. The report helps an RT set TR goals consistent with a lead doctor's treatment goals

71. When reporting an RT patient's progress, which of these is the most objective basis?

a. The RT's intuitive sense that the patient has improved
b. Comparison of current measures to baseline measures
c. Consensus on the treatment team of patient progress
d. The patient's self-report of experiencing improvement

72. The Measurable Assessment in Recreation for Resident-Centered Care (MARRCC) is designed for RTs working in long-term care settings and has four sections. Which section helps RTs to monitor changes in a resident's levels of functioning?

a. The Intake Assessment measuring function levels in four recreation-related domains
b. The Annual/Change of Condition/Re-admit Assessment for adjusting the TR program
c. The Care Plan Section to write measurable, problem-related, resident-centered goals
d. The Progress Note Section to evaluate resident progress and care plan effectiveness

73. Of the following concepts, which would be most related to enabling people with disabilities to participate in the same activities as the non-disabled in the same school class or community group?

a. TR/RT as inclusive recreation
b. TR/RT as treatment modality
c. TR/RT as a recreative process
d. TR/RT from holistic approach

74. Which of the following models of TR/RT features four steps and moves from maximum to minimum control by the therapist?

a. The Health Protection/Promotion model
b. The TR Service Delivery model
c. The Leisure Ability model
d. The Ecological model

75. Among the following psychology concepts, which one is most emphasized by the Health Protection/Health Promotion model of TR/RT?

a. Learned helplessness
b. Intrinsic motivation
c. Self-actualization
d. Locus of control

76. Of the following, which is a setting where RTs would NOT practice?

a. RTs may practice in all of these
b. In the public school systems
c. In psychiatric facilities
d. In clients' homes

77. Which of the following ATRA Standards for the Practice of TR is represented by a TR Department's providing its employees with opportunities for professional development?

a. Quality Management
b. Written Plan of Operation
c. Program Evaluation and Research
d. Staff Qualifications, Competency Assessment

78. RTs must provide prospective clients/patients with information that allows them to make decisions about accepting or declining treatment. To which principle of the ATRA Code of Ethics does this relate most?

a. Beneficence
b. Competence
c. Confidentiality
d. Informed Consent

79. If a practitioner of TR/RT very frequently cancels appointments with a client, which of the following is true?

a. This could violate the ATRA Code of Ethics Principle 6, Veracity
b. This would violate the ATRA Code of Ethics Principle 5, Fidelity
c. This reflects time management issues, not an ethical violation
d. This directly violates ATRA Ethics Principle 2, Non-Maleficence

80. For assessing a client/patient's physical functioning, which component reflects his/her relative ability to withstand exertion over periods of time?

a. Balance
b. Endurance
c. Activity level
d. Coordination

81. Assessment of which aspect of physical functioning is most closely associated with a person's flexibility for stretching and bending?

a. Strength
b. Wellness
c. Endurance
d. Coordination

82. Which of the following is most accurate about assessment in RT?

a. The vast majority of RTs routinely use standardized interviews to screen leisure history and interests
b. Client improvement cannot be measured without baselines measured by standardized assessments
c. Among RTs, most have a thorough education in standardized assessment tools for the practice of TR
d. RTs commonly assess specific functioning areas and targeted treatments utilizing standardized tools

83. What is true about the ATRA Standards for Practice regarding assessment of clients?

a. ATRA Standards for Practice do not specifically include anything on assessment
b. The ATRA only discusses assessment separately from its Standards for Practice
c. More than one ATRA Standard for Practice relates to assessment in some way
d. ATRA Standards for Practice are meant for treatment rather than assessment

84. Which of the following assessment instruments measures a client's functional skills?

a. Parts of the Idyll Arbor Leisure Battery
b. FOX Activity Therapy Skills Baseline
c. The CERT-Physical Disabilities
d. The CERT-PSYCH-R

85. What is true about the Therapeutic Recreation Activity Assessment (TRAA)?

a. It measures gross and fine motor skills, but does not assess social behaviors
b. None of these is true about the Therapeutic Recreation Activity Assessment
c. It tests motor skills and social behaviors, but it excludes communication skills
d. It measures motor, social, and communication skills but omits cognitive skills

86. If an assessment instrument can be repeated over time in multiple administrations and yield stable results, what does this mean statistically?

a. The instrument is reliable
b. The instrument is valid
c. It is reliable and valid
d. It is none of these

87. Which of the following is a definition of construct validity?

a. How well a test represents the entire subject or construct it tests
b. How well a test's current scores show what future scores will be
c. How well a test's scores relate to a similar test at the same time
d. How well a test measures an abstract idea (example: intelligence)

88. When a scientist statistically computes a correlation coefficient to assess the validity of a test instrument for measuring the thing it is meant to measure, what kind of validity is this?

a. Face validity
b. Construct validity
c. Predictive validity
d. Concurrent validity

89. Which kind of measurement errors will affect the reliability of a test?

a. Constant errors
b. Both of these
c. Random errors
d. Neither of these

90. Which type of reliability is most likely to be affected if the test-taker has grown older and/or learned more between administrations, and/or remembers material from taking the same test previously?

a. Inter-rater reliability
b. Test-retest reliability
c. Alternate-forms reliability
d. Internal consistency reliability

91. Which of the following kinds of test reliability is NOT established by computing correlation?

a. Rationale equivalence reliability
b. Equivalent-forms reliability
c. Test-retest reliability
d. Split-half reliability

92. If the RT selects an assessment that is very thorough and requires the test-taker to focus attention for long periods of time, and wants to administer it to a child who is young and/or diagnosed with ADHD, to which criterion for assessment selection does this relate?

a. Availability
b. Practicality
c. Reliability
d. Purpose

93. Related to assessment of a patient/client, which of the following would LEAST involve a behavioral observation?

a. The patient's amount and kinds of motor activity
b. The patient's body language and what it conveys
c. The patient's attention span in terms of its length
d. The patient's interpersonal and social interactions

94. The Ohio Scale of Leisure Functioning (OFA), the Comprehensive Evaluation for Recreational Therapy (CERT), and the Assessment of Characteristics of Therapeutic Recreation (FACTR) are examples of

a. leisure assessments.
b. functional assessments.
c. neurological assessments.
d. rehabilitation assessments.

95. The RT is testing a patient's awareness of danger and ability to care for himself or herself. In which functional domain does this part of the assessment belong?

a. Emotional
b. Cognitive
c. Sensory
d. Physical

96. A client finds leisure activity a way to escape from a stressful job. Which of the four primary leisure motivations does this reflect?

a. Competence mastery
b. Intellectual motivation
c. Stimulus avoidance
d. Social motivation

97. Which of these would likely be the RT's best source of assessment data for determining how many times a patient has had surgery for the same chronic condition affecting physical activity?

a. The family history
b. Family interviews
c. The medical charts
d. The team members

98. What has research shown about exercise therapy for patients with Multiple Sclerosis (MS)?

a. Exercise rehabilitation has been shown to exacerbate the symptoms for Multiple Sclerosis patients
b. Exercise rehabilitation has been shown to help physical and neurological function and quality of life
c. Exercise rehabilitation has been shown to increase the rates of relapse for Multiple Sclerosis clients
d. Exercise rehabilitation has been shown to reverse the progression of neurological impairment in MS

99. If a patient has a seizure disorder and displays poor coordination, an unsteady gait, slurred speech, confusion, and becomes aggressive, which of the following should the RT consider first?

a. These are common symptoms of alcohol and drug addictions
b. These are common side-effects of many seizure medications
c. These are common symptoms of certain mental health issues
d. These are common side-effects of having any seizure disorder

100. When interpreting the scores of a published standardized assessment, which of these is correct?

a. The scores must be interpreted via norm-referenced, not criterion-referenced methods
b. The scores must be interpreted using norm-referenced or criterion-referenced methods
c. The scores must be interpreted via criterion-referenced, not norm-referenced methods
d. The scores must be interpreted by the RT but need not be norm- or criterion-referenced

101. Which of the following assessment instruments would be most informative specifically for evaluating a patient's progress in treatment?

a. Measurement of Social Empowerment and Trust
b. The Leisure Satisfaction Measure
c. The Leisure Interest Measure
d. The Leisure Motivation Scale

102. In the Measurable Assessment in Recreation for Resident-Centered Care (MARRCC), the section called the Annual/Change of Condition/Re-Admit Assessment is most appropriate for which of these?

a. Adjustment of a care plan to meet changed resident needs
b. Evaluation of a resident's initial recreation-related functions
c. Evaluation of resident progress toward the care plan's goals
d. Assessment of the effectiveness of the individual care plan

103. A sentinel event is:

a. a sudden decline in patient satisfaction scores.
b. a local national disaster that requires implementation of the facility's emergency management plan.
c. a situation within a healthcare facility that places the employees and patients in a position of danger.
d. an unplanned incident within a healthcare facility that results in death or psychological damage to a patient.

104. A tool used to help organize and structure the plan for attaining goals is called:

a. constructive competence.
b. SMART goals.
c. continual service improvement goals.
d. feature advantage benefits.

105. Which of the following documentation tools would be most useful for the Recreation Therapist working at an inpatient rehabilitation facility?

a. FIM
b. SOAP
c. DARP
d. SOAPIER

106. The Recreation Therapist is completing a SOAP note on a patient who has recently been admitted for inpatient rehabilitation following a car accident. Which portion of the assessment would be documented in the "S" portion of the SOAP note?

a. Continue to encourage patient to attend the morning men's group daily
b. Patient was able to participate in the group activity without any limitations
c. Vital signs have been stable since admission
d. "My hands hurt so bad when I try to move my fingers."

107. In the SOAP method of charting, where would the RT place notes about the specific activities to use with a patient?

a. In the same place where the doctor notes the diagnosis
b. In the same place where prior treatments/providers are
c. In the same place where the doctor charts prescriptions
d. In the same place where a patient pain rating is charted

108. The RT is reading in a chart the date when a patient stated they sustained an injury and how it happened. According to the SOAP method of documentation, where would this note be entered?

a. In the "S" section
b. In the "O" section
c. In the "A" section
d. In the "P" section

109. The Functional Independence Measure (FIM) contains how many total items?

a. 36
b. 18
c. 07
d. 30

110. Which of the following is true about the Functional Independence Measure (FIM)?

a. It has been statistically found reliable but not found to be valid
b. It has been statistically found valid but not found to be reliable
c. It is particularly specific to diagnoses of traumatic brain injuries (TBI)
d. It identifies patient changes during inpatient rehabilitation programs

111. The Functional Independence Measure (FIM) is designed for evaluating the areas of dysfunction that people experience in activities when they have which kinds of disorders?

a. Reversible, permanent, or progressive, neurologic, musculoskeletal, and others
b. Permanent, reversible, or progressive; and musculoskeletal but not neurological
c. Musculoskeletal and neurological; permanent and reversible but not progressive
d. Progressive and permanent, not reversible; neurological but not musculoskeletal

112. In an outdoor RT program for teens with psychiatric, emotional, behavior, and/or addiction disorders, which of the following is the best example of a behavioral objective?

a. "The client will demonstrate the ability to climb inside of a cave in a safe manner."
b. "When asked, the client will climb in a cave using the climbing technique as taught."
c. "When inside of a cave, the client will know the proper climbing technique to use."
d. "The client will understand the proper techniques to use for climbing inside caves."

113. The results of the US Census for 2021 show that which of the following leisure activities was done the most by both males and females in terms of daily hours spent?

a. Playing games and using the computer
b. Exercising
c. Socializing
d. Watching TV

114. In making an activity analysis to choose RT activities for an individual client, which example is the most appropriate choice?

a. Playing games of tag for a client goal to follow directions in sequence
b. Building a birdhouse for a client goal to follow directions in sequence
c. Building a birdhouse for a client goal to improve skills for socialization
d. Playing basketball toward a client goal to improve skills for socializing

115. Which facilitation technique would be most appropriate for the RT to use for crafts with a client who has motor apraxia?

a. Reality therapy
b. Hand-over-hand
c. Step sequencing
d. Cognitive reframing

116. For people with disabilities who are wheelchair-bound, which recreational activity is most likely to involve additional assistive computer technology?

a. Reading books
b. Creative writing
c. Going to movies
d. Watching the TV

117. In the long-term care setting, at what point during the day do residents often show more signs of agitation?

a. When they are not occupied with an activity
b. In the middle of the night
c. At lunch time
d. During medication administrations

118. A 21-year-old complete spinal cord injury patient is apprehensive about attending a support group for those who have suffered this type of injury. The RT is explaining some of the positive benefits of participating, one of which is:

a. finding who he can blame for his situation.
b. meeting members of the opposite sex to start dating again.
c. finding solutions to problems he is having adapting from those who have gone through the same process.
d. verbalizing his feelings when he is required to do so during that portion of the meeting.

119. Which of the following behavior modification techniques would be most helpful for a client with agoraphobia?

a. Differential reinforcement of incompatible behavior (DRI)
b. Differential reinforcement of other behavior (DRO)
c. Systematic desensitization
d. Positive reinforcement

120. In which of the following ways has leisure counseling been identified as a valuable psychotherapeutic tool?

a. Researchers have identified all of these as applications of leisure counseling
b. Easing symptoms of phobias, panic attacks, or post-traumatic stress disorder
c. Controlling and/or inhibiting obsessive, compulsive, and addictive behaviors
d. Helping patients in establishing and maintaining positive moods and feelings

121. Relative to the nature and diversity of recreation and leisure activities, what element is LEAST important for RTs to include in their programs to promote their advocacy for all kinds of people?

a. Activities that make us examine biases
b. Activities that make us examine phobias
c. Activities that make us examine prejudices
d. Activities that make us examine disease etiology.

122. A device that can help stroke rehabilitation patients to improve range of motion and function in the hands is:

a. a finger contracture orthotic.
b. a Smart Glove.
c. a resting hand splint.
d. a terry cloth hand cone.

123. A 72-year-old female has sustained a stroke which has caused her to have right-sided hemiplegia. She has speech problems with forming words, problems with dressing and bathing due to the hemiplegia, and is developing contractures in her right hand. Considering the problems she now has with day-to-day life, which of the following would be considered a problem with performing instrumental ADLs?

a. Dressing
b. Bathing
c. Housekeeping
d. Brushing teeth

124. A 37-year-old male sustained bilateral lower leg amputations after a work-related accident. He has healed physically, and would like to try to get back in the work force. He had worked as a construction worker but is not able to perform those duties now. Which resource would be the most helpful to him?

a. Physical therapy
b. Speech therapy
c. Occupational therapy
d. Vocation rehabilitation

125. Which of the following is the responsibility of the referring provider in a consultation?

a. Explain to the patient the purpose for a consultation and the name of the consulting provider
b. Contact the patient's insurance carrier to request a peer-to-peer review for any future treatment
c. Inform the patient that they will need to seek the services of a provider within a certain specialty on their own
d. Wait for a request for records and any diagnostic testing that has been completed

126. When teaching a patient who has a hearing impairment, it is important to:

a. face them directly so one's face and lips are clearly visible to them.
b. give them educational materials in print to take home and read on their own.
c. have the patient be the only person receiving educational material so they can feel more involved in their treatment plan.
d. discuss the treatment plan with the spouse or family so that they can communicate with the patient in the way that best suits his needs.

127. Four components of TR program design are: Purpose, Population, Process, and Setting. Which of the following lists the meaning or content of each of these in the same order as they are listed above?

a. Who, What, Where, and How
b. Where, What, Why, and Who
c. When, Why, Who, and How
d. Why, Who, How, and Where

128. The Recreation Therapist is helping a patient and her family with some of her rehabilitative needs upon discharge. She would like to continue Recreation Therapy because it has been helpful with the physical and psychological effects of multiple sclerosis, but she lives in a rural area where Recreation Therapy is not readily available. She has Medicare for her primary insurance. She is inquiring about receiving this service via a telehealth service. The RT's best response is:

a. that they will request the physician order this and it can be set up for her.
b. a Recreation Therapist can come to her home and perform the services there.
c. she will have to return to the rehabilitation facility for Recreation Therapy services.
d. Recreation Therapy services are rarely available via telehealth, but it is hoped they will be in the future.

129. Under which category does recreation therapy fall?

a. Analytic therapy
b. Experiential therapy
c. Psychological therapy
d. Psychiatric therapy

130. TR services can be included in health care services, leisure services, educational services, and transition services. In which two is the RT most likely to use the APIE process for designing specific interventions and programs rather than an IEP or an ITP?

a. Transition services and health care services
b. Education services and transition services
c. Health care services and leisure services
d. Leisure services and education services

131. Which of the following is NOT classified as an axis in service delivery systems?

a. Public-Private
b. Profit-Nonprofit
c. Clinical-Community
d. Health-Human Services

132. Which of the following is one of the purposes for developing the Prospective Payment System (PPS) for health care services, which can include RT services?

a. The PPS sets, but does not limit, costs
b. The PPS is unrelated to service quality
c. The PPS excludes Medicare recipients
d. The PPS creates client-centered focus

133. Regarding documentation of assessments, functional status, profess, discharge plans, and transition plans for a client, which of the following is accurate about Source-Oriented Medical Records (SOMRs) and Problem-Oriented Medical Records (POMRs)?

a. A SOMR is organized into a data base, a problem list, an initial plan, and progress notes
b. A POMR is organized into a data base, a problem list, an initial plan, and progress notes
c. A POMR divides charts into disciplines with medical notes, nursing notes, TR notes, etc.
d. A SOMR and a POMR both include all seven of the sections named in the other choices

134. Which of these correctly represents some things that RTs should consider when evaluating their TR programs?

a. If results are good, the program's role is immaterial
b. Efficacy of the program, not relative activity efficacy
c. Implementation's effectiveness, not its correctness
d. A costs-to-benefits analysis of the program's results

135. The purpose of quality improvement is to:

a. improve employee satisfaction.
b. monitor the leadership skills of the administration of a healthcare facility.
c. implement specific changes in healthcare which have a measurable improvement for a group of patients.
d. provide specific training and education opportunities to employees to ensure the quality of the care provided is reaching high standards.

136. What is accurate about utilization review as a part of quality improvement?

a. Utilization review concentrates on over-utilization, not under-utilization
b. Utilization review concentrates on under-utilization, not over-utilization
c. Utilization review targets department inefficiency but not effectiveness
d. Utilization review should be included in written agency operations plans

137. In planning a TR program, which of the following involves operational units found among the resources that RT personnel have available, which can be used in program implementation to fulfill some parts of their mission statement and comprehensive program goals?

a. The analysis
b. The investigation
c. The determination
d. The conceptualization

138. Which of the following accurately reflects NCTRC requirements for supervisors of TR/RT internships?

a. At a university, a supervisor must have been a CTRS for one year to supervise interns
b. At an agency, the supervisor must have been a CTRS for one year to supervise interns
c. At an agency, the supervisor must be employed there a minimum of 25 hours a week
d. At an agency, a supervisor of internships must have 25% of job duties in a TR program

139. An example of a third-party payer is:

a. the patient.
b. the patient's employer.
c. a health insurance company.
d. a worker's compensation coverage company.

140. The medical service that is covered under Medicare Part A is:

a. Laboratory tests.
b. Appointments with a primary care provider.
c. Appointments with a specialist.
d. Prescription drug coverage.

141. Which of the following is true about Medicare and Medicaid?

a. Both Medicare and Medicaid provide health insurance only for those aged 65 and over
b. Medicare is a federal program and Medicaid is a combined federal and state program
c. Medicare Part A provides for hospital care, home health care, and outpatient services
d. Medicare Part B provides for hospital care, home health care, and outpatient services

142. Which of these is accurate regarding budgeting for TR/RT facilities?

a. A TR/RT facility's operating budget defines daily expenses and revenues
b. A TR/RT facility's capital expenditure budget covers a period of one year
c. A TR/RT facility's revenue and expense budget usually covers 3 to 5 years
d. A TR/RT facility's capital expenditure budget specifies its everyday costs

143. What is true of the Joint Commission, CARF, and other groups regulating TR/RT accreditation relative to NCTRC?

a. The NCTRC has better relationships with the Joint Commission and CARF via its association with NTRS and ATRA
b. The NCTRC has better relationships with the Joint Commission and CARF via independence from NTRS and ATRA
c. The NCTRC provides the same credentials for TR/RT that are provided by the Joint Commission and CARF
d. The NCTRC provides TR/RT credentials, including certification as well as registration and licensure

144. Regarding professional development for the RT, which is accurate about continuing education?

a. Attending webinars and teleconferences is not approved as attending class in person is
b. RTs can earn up to 25 continuing education credits for presentations and/or publications
c. RTs cannot use their academic theses or dissertations to earn continuing education units
d. 1 Continuing Education Unit (CEU) is equivalent to 1 credit, or 1 educational contact hour

145. Which statement is most accurate regarding regulations in the USA to practice TR/RT?

a. Requirements of all states in the USA are uniformly governed by Federal regulations
b. Every state in the USA requires RTs to have both licensure and certification to practice
c. A minimum of a Bachelor's degree is generally required, but regulations vary by state
d. A license to practice RT is required by only a few US states, but all require certification

146. How can a RT working within an agency best promote a TRS program's value?

a. Through regular reports of progress to administrators
b. Through the publication of articles in academic journals
c. Through making presentations to groups of volunteers
d. Through participation in professional groups' meetings

147. Which of the following is true regarding the American Therapeutic Recreation Association (ATRA)?

a. There are larger national organizations for TR than ATRA
b. Less than ¼ of the CTRSs in the country belong to ATRA
c. More RTs belong to ATRA than OTs belonging to AOTA
d. ATRA has a PAC with similar funding to the AOTA PAC

148. What is one way the NCTRC ensures that the continuing education pursued by CTRSs contributes value to the advancement of the TR/RT profession?

a. By giving CTRSs CEUs or credits for every continuing education experience they complete
b. By requiring their CE experiences to be connected to knowledge areas in the Job Analysis
c. By offering its own series of continuing education courses online in which CTRSs can enroll
d. By providing continuing education via home study courses and professional journal review

149. Which of the following is true regarding provider-patient boundaries?

a. It is acceptable for a provider's involvement with a patient to extend into personal or business relationships
b. It is reasonable to believe that the recreational therapist, as the patient's provider, is the only one who really understands the patient or who can help the patient
c. It is appropriate to divert personal questions the patient has about oneself or one's family back to the patient to focus the attention on the patient's problems
d. It is appropriate to meet with a patient somewhere outside of work to discuss any problems they are having

150. The Recreation Therapist is riding in the elevator with a co-worker at the end of their shift, along with a few hospital visitors. She is complaining about the very demanding parents of one of the patients she cared for today. The most appropriate response from the co-worker is to:

a. try to lighten the mood and make her feel better after a hard shift.
b. quietly let her know she should not be discussing patient care in a public place.
c. tell her about some difficulty patients they had to care for during their shift, also.
d. say nothing, but report the conversation to the Risk Management Department at the hospital.

Answer Key and Explanations

1. C: Piaget and researchers following him have found that most people typically reach the stage of Formal Operations, wherein they can perform mental operations without using concrete objects, by the pre-teen or early teen years. Young children do not achieve this, let alone infants (A). Though it is possible, it is unusual for an individual not to develop this cognitive skill until early (B) or middle adulthood (D).

2. D: Psychologist Abraham Maslow developed a 5-level hierarchy of human needs. The most basic are the needs for safety and protection of life, followed by being loved and belonging to a social group. These are followed by a feeling of accomplishment and self-esteem. The highest level in Maslow's hierarchy is achieving self-actualization, when a person reaches their full potential and has mastered the lower levels.

3. B: The brain of a newborn infant typically weighs around 25% of what it will weigh in adulthood. Babies' brains do not weigh half as much (A) as adults' brains, let alone ¾ as much (D). But they weigh more than twice as much as only 10% (C) of what they will weigh when the babies have become adults.

4. B: The 1-1/2 to 3-year-old child is starting to make their own decisions by walking away from a parent or choosing which toy to play with or food he would like to eat. Erikson has called this second stage of development a period during which the child experiences autonomy vs. shame and doubt when they begin to exercise their independence.

5. D: From mature adulthood (old age) to death, Erikson found that people review their lives and either feel mainly fulfillment and wisdom, or sorrow/bitterness and despair. He termed this period and its nuclear conflict that of Ego Integrity vs. Despair. Erikson called adolescence (A) the period and conflict of Identity vs. Role Confusion, when teens succeed or fail at establishing sense of self and personal identity. He termed young adulthood (B) the period and crisis of Intimacy vs. Isolation, when people succeed or fail at forging close relationships with others. He called middle adulthood (C) the period and conflict of Generativity vs. Stagnation, when people create and/or cultivate legacies for the future, such as children and other accomplishments that will outlive them.

6. A: Skinner was a major proponent and developer of behaviorism, the theory that we learn by responding to environmental stimuli with observable behaviors; and that what consequences occur as results of, or immediately following, our behaviors shape our subsequent behaviors. Freud (B) attributed human behavior to unconscious impulses, governed by drives toward sex and death, and personality defense mechanisms, etc. Gardner (C) did not explain human behavior but studied human intelligence, and theorized that there are multiple (nine) different types or forms of intelligence related to different domains. Maslow (D) attributed human behavior to fulfilling needs he organized into a hierarchy, from the most basic physical needs to the highest self-actualization needs, whose fulfillment he said was necessarily progressive.

7. B: Albert Bandura, who proposed Social Learning Theory, coined the term self-efficacy to define specifically a person's belief in his/her competence to achieve a goal. Humanist psychologist Carl Rogers coined the term the actualizing tendency (A) to define that life force that is the innate motivation to develop one's potentials to the fullest. A humanist like Rogers, Maslow coined the term self-actualization (C) to define not only the full development of one's potentials, but the highest level of need in his hierarchy of needs. Industry was part of the developmental stage and nuclear conflict that psychosocial theorist Erikson (D) named Industry vs. Inferiority. Successfully resolving this conflict does result in a general feeling of one's overall competence as a person, according to Erikson. Bandura's self-efficacy is a more specific sense of competence that one can accomplish an outcome.

8. C: Humanistic psychologist Carl Rogers coined the terms "person-centered" and "client-centered" therapy to name the type of treatment he practiced and advocated. Of the choices given, his legacy has most contributed to the person-centered model of health and human services. Because he emphasized the role of community in creating meaning, Vygotsky (A) can be said to have contributed to community models of health and human services. While Erikson (B) did not work directly with rehabilitation, his theory of personality development is a psychosocial one that emphasizes the individual's relationship to society; so it generally contributes most to the psychosocial rehabilitation model in that this model focuses on the individual's functioning in society. Kraus & Shank (D) are among those proposing various medical or clinical models, which have contributed most to the traditional medical model of H&HS that views client needs as illnesses to be treated.

9. A: The educational and/or training model of H&HS, including TR, is most often followed with developmentally disabled populations. It emphasizes acquiring skills needed to contribute to society, including social skills and leisure skills. It is often used in special education schools, vocational rehabilitation centers, sheltered workshops, and daycare settings. The psychosocial rehabilitation (B) model is more often used for clients with severe and chronic mental illnesses rather than with developmental disabilities. This model promotes optimal community functioning, including activity participation. The recovery model (C) is adapted from the model for recovery from substance abuse and is used for both addictions and serious mental illnesses. The community model (D) emphasizes providing a broader range of community-based opportunities for leisure activities and the skills to participate in them.

10. B: The ICF classifies both health and disability, according to the World Health Organization (WHO), which created the ICF. The WHO states that the ICF supports its aim to shift the approach from viewing health vs. disability as separate categories, to viewing various levels of health and how these affect people's functioning. Thus, the ICF reflects the WHO's vision that health is not an absence of disability (A); and that disability is not a lack of health (C), but that all levels of health are included in this common measurement of how people function in society. The WHO finds that emphasizing effects instead of causes "...places all health conditions on an equal footing..." Functioning is not a direct measure of the ICF, therefore, (D) is incorrect.

11. D: The planning and development of resources, such as what RT, healthcare, and other services a client will need, is an example of how the ICF can be applied for providing services at the institutional level. Communicating with other practitioners; healthcare, social service, and community agencies (A) is an example of how the ICF can be used at the individual level. Making needs assessments of a client's limitations or restrictions in participating in activities (B) is an example of how the ICF can be used at the social level, as is making environmental assessments for universal design (C).

12. A: As of the 2020 Census, the state with the highest diversity index remains Hawaii (which was also the case in 2010). The largest ethnic group of the state of California is the Hispanic/Latino population (making up about 39% of a very diversely populated state) and the largest ethnic group of the District of Columbia is Black/African American (making up about 41% of the population). Overall, the Hispanic/Latino population remains the largest minority group across the country, making up about 19% of the total population.

13. C: In order to become a certified Recreational Therapist, the candidate must first obtain a Bachelor's Degree in Recreational Therapy or a related field. A supervised internship that offers at least 560 hours must also be completed, as well as successfully pass the certification exam. A Master's Degree in Recreational Therapy is also available to achieve a higher level of education and training.

14. B: Cultural encounter is the process of encouraging medical staff to interact with those patients who are from a different cultural background. It has been found that the more a person interacts with those from different cultures, the more their beliefs and practices can be understood. Communities have become very diverse and the medical professional needs to be prepared to address the individual needs and practices of those from different cultures.

15. A: According to a popular theoretical model (Wheeler, 1994) for the cultural diversity training of RTs, there are four levels of cultural competency. The lowest is unconsciously incompetent (C), meaning therapists do not know what they do not know about cultural diversity, and are unaware of their own cultural prejudices, biases, stereotypes, and reactions to diverse clients. The second level is consciously incompetent (B), meaning the therapists have inadequate cultural knowledge and sensitivity, but are aware of their own cultural biases and values and are motivated to increase their cultural understanding and effectiveness. The third level is consciously competent (D), meaning the therapists have and apply awareness and comprehension of cultural diversity in implementing TR programs. The fourth and highest level is unconsciously competent (A), meaning therapists know how to provide culturally competent TR services, and do so naturally without having to think about it.

16. B: The systems theory concept of homeostasis means that groups tend to behave in ways that promote equilibrium, regularity, and safety. When a group develops its own rules in addition to those the therapist has provided, and those rules keep the group system stable, this reflects the tendency toward homeostasis. How members share or exclude information within the group, and how they accept or reject and process that information (A) reflects the systems theory concept of group information exchange. Whether feedback within a group provokes conflict resulting in changes to the system (C) reflects the systems theory concept that positive feedback tends to change the system while negative feedback resists change and tends to support the system status quo. The interdependence of group members (D) reflects the systems theory concept that a group is a holistic entity, i.e. greater than the sum of its parts, rather than a collection of single individuals.

17. A: Neuropsychological assessment (and also psychiatric evaluation in some cases) must be conducted for differentially diagnosing the symptoms named, because all of these symptoms can exist in cases of intellectual disability (B), aphasia and similar language disorders (C), or dementia (D); therefore, any of these conditions (as well as delirium, encephalopathy, or pseudodementia secondary to mental illness or substance abuse) can be confused because of the similar symptoms.

18. B: Patients with an injury at the C5 level will require assistance with most of the activities of daily living. With training, though, they should be able to operate a power wheelchair on their own. These patients will have partial or total paralysis of the wrists, hands, trunk and legs, but may be able to raise their arms and bend their elbows. Breathing may be weakened, but they are still able to speak and use the diaphragm. Injuries higher than the C5 level have a greater impact on breathing and functioning of the arms and hands.

19. A: The Individuals with Disabilities Education Act (IDEA) was signed into law to ensure that all children have access to an appropriate education despite their disabilities. It also ensures that special education services are available to children. This was originally known as the Education of

Handicapped Children Act, which was put into place in 1975. It was updated, amended, and the name changed to IDEA in 1990.

20. D: MS affects the nervous system and can cause muscle atrophy and restrict the patient's flexibility and range of motion, among other symptoms, so ROM activities are especially important. TR activities to strengthen the muscles are especially important for patients with Spina Bifida (A), which can cause varying degrees of paralysis. TR activities that encourage movement to maintain muscle tone are especially important for patients with Muscular Dystrophy (B), which causes progressive wasting of the muscular tissues. TR activities involving use of gross motor skills are especially important for patients with Cerebral Palsy (C), which causes difficulty with control and coordination of muscular movements.

21. D: A stroke to the brain's left hemisphere can impair the patient's language and memory, so using physical gestures, demonstrations, and modeling will be more effective than verbal instructions. Leisure education is more appropriate for patients who have had right-hemisphere strokes, which can impair visual, spatial and depth perception; reality orientation is more likely needed for patients with left-hemisphere strokes, which more often impair emotional processing and social interactions (A). Removing distractions from the environment (B) is more important for patients with right-hemisphere strokes because their perception of their surroundings is more likely impaired. These patients are also more likely to respond better to verbal directions than patients with left-hemisphere strokes, not vice versa (C).

22. B: Phenylketonuria is a metabolic disorder wherein the body cannot process trace amounts of copper in foods. Type 1 Diabetes mellitus (A), Cushing syndrome (C), and hyperthyroidism (D) are all categorized as endocrine disorders. In metabolic disorders, the body cannot adequately process nutrients; whereas in endocrine disorders, certain hormones are not adequately produced by the glands. In Type 1 diabetes, the pancreas produces insufficient insulin. In Cushing syndrome, the adrenal glands produce excessive cortisol—or this excess develops from taking corticosteroid medication for too long. In hyperthyroidism, the thyroid gland produces too much thyroxine, a thyroid hormone.

23. A: Infectious diseases can be contracted by humans through three kinds of direct contact: Human-to-human; animal-to-human; and mother-to-unborn baby. They can be transmitted by indirect contact, as when touching anything that an infected person has previously touched; hence (B) and (D) are incorrect. They can be contracted through the bites of insects, such as ticks, mosquitoes, fleas, or lice. And they can also be transmitted through contaminated food and/or water, as with E. coli bacteria, salmonella (including typhoid fever), Giardia, dysentery, hepatitis A, etc.; hence (C) is incorrect.

24. A: Otitis media is an infection of the middle ear that can cause fluid buildup in the middle ear space, and if untreated can result in a ruptured eardrum from the pressure. Any hearing loss caused in the outer or middle ear is conductive, i.e. something impedes the conduction of sound waves to the inner ear; and is often reversible/partially reversible. Sensorineural (B) hearing loss is caused in the inner ear, nerves, and/or brain. For example, when the hair cells in the cochlea of the inner ear die or are destroyed, sound impulses cannot be transmitted to the auditory/acoustic nerve and thence the brain. Damage to the auditory nerve and/or the brain's auditory processing centers also causes sensorineural hearing loss, which is permanent and irreversible. (Cochlear implants can restore hearing in some cases of cochlear damage/defect.) Mixed hearing loss (C) is a combination of (A) and (B), which would not be caused *only* by otitis media. Therefore, (D) is incorrect.

25. A: Strabismus is a condition wherein the muscles of both eyes do not work together. Nystagmus (B) is a condition of involuntary, repetitive eye movements. Presbyopia (C) is the type of farsightedness that develops due to aging, as the ability of the eyes to focus at nearer distances decreases. Retinopathy (D) is a condition of damage or defect in the light-sensitive retina, which normally sends images to the brain via the optic nerve. Diabetes causes vascular changes that can result in diabetic retinopathy; and premature infants can suffer from retinopathy of prematurity (ROP), previously called retrolental fibroplasia.

26. A: The terminology of the diagnosis for obsessive-compulsive disorder refers to obsessive thinking, i.e. constantly and repetitively dwelling involuntarily on the same anxieties, worries, fears, or needs; and compulsive doing, i.e. constantly and repetitively performing actions in response to the obsessive thoughts. Choice (B) has the meaning reversed. Choice (C) is also backwards: ritualistic behaviors are the compulsive component and are responses to fixations, which are obsessive, rather than vice versa. These terms do not refer to both obsessiveness and compulsiveness of both thinking and doing (D): obsession is mental and compulsion is physical.

27. B: One sign of drug abuse is getting into trouble with the law because of it, e.g. getting arrested for driving under the influence of alcohol or other drugs, for stealing to support an addiction, for disorderly conduct, etc. However, this is not necessarily a sign of drug addiction. If a person has developed a tolerance to the drug of choice; i.e. s/he needs larger amounts of it to get the same effects as from smaller quantities before (A), this is a sign of drug addiction. So is a need to take the drug of choice to relieve or prevent withdrawal symptoms (C), e.g. depression, anxiety, restlessness, insomnia, shaking, sweating, nausea, etc. Loss of control over how much and/or how often one uses (D) the drug(s), even if one wants to quit or control use, is another sign of addiction.

28. A: According to the Title I statute of the IDEA (Individuals with Disabilities Education Act), children with disabilities are entitled to a free, appropriate public education (FAPE) in the least restrictive environment (LRE), meaning that unless the severity and/or nature of a child's disability makes it impossible, children with disabilities are to be educated in regular schools and classes together with non-disabled children. This includes providing supplementary services and supports that will enable children with disabilities to have such an education. This statute regards special classes (B) or separate schools (C) as NOT the LRE for children with disabilities (unless mainstreamed education "cannot be achieved satisfactorily", even with supplementary services). However, IDEA stipulates that giving children with disabilities the supplementary services they need to succeed in regular classes is part of the LRE, rather than deeming such added services restrictive (D).

29. C: The Rehabilitation Act of 1973 protects individuals with disabilities from discrimination. The Access Board, which enforces the Architectural Barriers Act to keep architectural barriers from preventing access to buildings by people with disabilities, was established under Section 502 of the Rehabilitation Act. Section 502 specifically prohibits federally funded facilities from having architectural, transportation, and communication barriers to disabled persons. Section 504 (D) of this law specifically prohibits federally funded entities from denying or excluding individuals with disabilities from equal opportunities to receive program services and benefits. Title III of the 2001 No Child Left Behind Act (A) requires federally funded schools to provide language instruction to students learning English as a second language (ESL) and/or with limited English-language proficiency (LEP). Title I of the NCLB Act (B) provides funding for educational services to school districts and schools in low-income areas whose students are economically and educationally disadvantaged.

30. A: These are all examples of stereotypes that many people in our society tend to believe. Stereotypes are not only negative, as when Americans think all Asian people in our country are always terrible drivers (D); they are also positive, as when white Americans think all African-Americans are athletically superior (B) or all Asian people are naturally more intelligent (C). While some highly publicized sports organizations like the NBA and the NFL include many African-American athletes, African-Americans like Tiger Woods (who is, like many identified as African-American, really multiracial - Black, White, Native American, Thai and Chinese) are in the minority among professional golfers. Not all African-Americans are athletically superior; a combination of higher visibility for those who are and cultural emphasis on athletic achievement is more realistic. All Asian people are not naturally more intelligent; rather, their culture places greater value on education and academic achievement.

31. B: The Americans with Disabilities Act (A) was most recently amended in 2008, effective in 2009. While the IDEA (A) or IDEIA (Individuals with Disabilities Education Improvement Act) had its last complete reauthorization in 2004, Part C of this law was updated with regulations for an early intervention program to serve children from birth to 2 years old in 2011. This was a partial but important update to prepare special-needs children for preschool and school. The Older Americans Act (C) was most recently amended in 2006. Therefore, (D) is incorrect as no two of these laws were updated most recently in the same year.

32. A: A number of states have laws regulating TR/RT or physical and occupational therapy. Some examples are the Oklahoma Therapeutic Recreation Practice Act; the North Carolina Recreational Therapy Licensure Act; the New Hampshire Statute (Title XXX, Occupations and Professions, Chapter 326-J, Recreational Therapists); and the Utah Administrative Code R156-40, Recreational Therapy Practice Act Rule. Also, Tennessee has a statute regulating physical and occupational therapy practices. Therefore, (B) is incorrect as not only the Federal government (e.g. the US Department of Labor) regulates TR/RT; (C) is incorrect as some states in the US do have laws regulating RT/TR; and (D) is incorrect as not all states currently have such regulations yet, although the NCTRC does advocate for it.

33. B: Aristotle proposed that leisure occurs on three different levels: the level of contemplation (A), the level of recreation (C), and the level of amusement (D). Perceived freedom (B) is a modern concept meaning freedom from obligations in order to engage in leisure activities, and freedom to choose and engage in activities without others' control; it can also refer to the modern paradox that though we perceive having freedom while engaging in leisure activities, in reality we are not truly free because there are always obligations that would eliminate any free time if we chose to meet all of them.

34. A: Recreation is defined by many experts as not only something we engage in during our free time, as leisure (B) is; and not only something enjoyable done for its inherent pleasure, as play (C) is; but moreover is morally acceptable, not just to the individual but also to the whole of society, and contributes to society in socially acceptable ways. Therefore, not all (D) of these fit that description.

35. A: "Balance" leisure activities are those that balance people's lives by providing them with more variety among recreational pursuits. Balance leisure activities also change throughout a person's life, while core leisure activities tend to remain more constant for an individual (B). Core leisure activities tend to cost less overall than balance activities (C) and be more accessible (D) as well.

36. C: The literature from research into leisure behavior has established that people tend to pursue roughly equivalent proportions of stability and novelty in their leisure activities. Adults have been found to have started approximately half of their leisure activities during childhood. Since they begin the other half in their later lives, this reflects that they seek stability about half of the time by continuing activities started in childhood; and novelty about half of the time by taking up new leisure experiences later on in their lives. Therefore, people do not prefer either stability (A) or novelty (B) in leisure; and seeking new leisure experiences is no more associated with youth than continuing familiar ones is with old age is (D).

37. C: The holistic approach to TR/RT places the most emphasis on considering each individual as a whole person and all addressing all the combined needs of that unique individual. The concept of TR/RT as a recreative experience (A) puts more emphasis on exposing participants to various types of experiences in recreation and assuring everybody a right to recreation. Special or adaptive recreation (B) focuses on how TR/RT can benefit people with disabilities or special needs, including the use of adaptive equipment and/or other accommodations or modifications in therapeutic techniques and routines as necessary to enable participation. TR/RT as a treatment modality (D) places more emphasis on using TR/RT to treat a specific illness or condition rather than emphasizing the whole person as holistic approaches do.

38. C: Community Inclusion services enable people with disabilities to participate in the same community TR/RT activities as people without disabilities by providing whatever adaptations, accommodations, and supports they need to do so. As such, it can encompass the specialty areas of physical medicine and rehabilitation (A), which applies TR/RT as part of treatment of various medical, physiological diseases, impairments, and conditions; developmental disabilities (B), which applies TR/RT as part of remediation of disabilities having onsets before adulthood; and behavioral health (D), which applies TR/RT as part of treatment for various disorders that affect emotional, cognitive, and behavioral functioning.

39. C: The Long-Term Care model (formerly the Custodial model) aims to maintain the functioning of people with chronic impairments at their optimal levels rather than to increase their functioning over time. The Treatment (or Medical) models and the Leisure Ability model (B) follow a continuum wherein the therapist helps the participant gradually gain higher levels of functioning and more independence in engaging in recreational activities. The Activity Therapy model (D) is like the Treatment or Medical models in that a doctor prescribes TR/RT, and therapy progresses on a continuum; its main difference is that it tends to include multiple therapeutic areas like art therapy, occupational therapy, music therapy, dance therapy, etc.

40. C: The Long-Term Care (formerly Custodial) model is most applied in practice settings like group homes, institutions, prisons, and nursing homes. Its focus is to maintain maximal health and wellbeing for chronically impaired persons rather than to rehabilitate. The Medical/Clinical model (A) focuses on treatment rather than overall client needs and is most applied in hospitals and in other medical and rehabilitation facilities. The Milieu Therapy model (B) emphasizes the client's environment and interactions with it and is most applied in mental health facilities. The Education/Training model (D) emphasizes teaching skills needed in society (e.g. leisure skills and social skills) and is most applied in schools, vocational rehabilitation centers, daycare centers, and sheltered workshops.

41. C: This is an example of ATRA's Standard 1 of Practice, Assessment. Standard 2, Treatment Planning (A), is concerned with developing an individualized treatment plan identifying goals, objectives, and specific intervention strategies AFTER the RT has conducted an individualized assessment by gathering comprehensive data about the client/patient. Standard 7, Ethical Conduct (B), is concerned with adhering to the ATRA Code of Ethics. Standard 5, Discharge Planning (D), concerns collaboration by the RT with the client/patient, family, and other members of the treatment team for continuing treatment as needed beyond discharge from a treatment facility.

42. B: Principle 4 of the ATRA Code of Ethics, Justice, reflects this. Principle 5, Fidelity (A), reflects the obligation of RTs to meet commitments to clients foremost, as well as secondarily to co-workers, agencies, and their profession. Principle 6, Veracity (C) reflects the requirement that RTs be honest and truthful. Principle 3, Autonomy (D) reflects the duty of RTs to protect client rights to choose in their own care plans, or to respect the decisions of legal representatives of clients unable to choose.

43. C: Principle 2, Nonmaleficence, stipulates that RTs have an obligation to help persons while respecting their decisions and protecting them from harm; Principle 5, Fidelity (A) stipulates that an RT's first obligation is to meet the commitments made to the person receiving services, and his/her second obligation is to their workplace and the profession; Principle 10, Compliance with Laws and Regulations (B) stipulates that RTs are responsible to comply with federal, state, and local laws, regulations, and ATRA policies concerning the RT profession, but does not mention protection from harm; Principle 6, Veracity (D) stipulates that RT's always be truthful and honest.

44. C: The ATRA Code of Ethics' Principle 6, Veracity, not only enjoins RT personnel to avoid telling untruths, but also to avoid "omitting what is true". Therefore, (A) is incorrect that this would violate none of the principles of this Code. Principle 5, Fidelity (B) pertains to loyalty and faithfulness to one's clients, as well as to the profession and one's colleagues, rather than to honesty and truthfulness. Principle 4, Justice (D) pertains to delivering services equitably without discrimination.

45. A: The psychosocial domain involves how the person functions psychologically and socially. The affective (B) domain involves the person's mood and/or emotional state. The cognitive (C) domain involves how the person functions intellectually. The physical (C) domain involves how the person functions bodily and in the environment.

46. B: The affective domain entails the person's emotional status and mood. Assessing it includes observing body language, facial expressions, and estimating self-esteem. Assessing the psychosocial (A) domain involves the person's self-concept or sense of self; his/her independence, capacity for developing relationships, engagement and interactions; dress and hygiene; etiquette, manners and other social behaviors; and demonstrations of competence, confidence, and degree of social anxiety if any. The cognitive (C) domain includes the person's learning capacity and processes; ability to attend and attention span; short-term memory; and ability to concentrate, follow directions, make decisions, and solve problems. The physical (D) domain includes the person's overall health and wellness; coordination, activity level, strength and flexibility; balance, and endurance.

47. D: The Comprehensive Evaluation in Recreational Therapy, or CERT, assessment is used in the short-term, acute care, psychiatric setting. In evaluates patients based on three areas of observation: general, individual performance, and group performance. The STIAP assessment is used with adults with physical disabilities and the MDS assessment is used for residents in nursing homes. The LBI assessment measures leisure barriers in 8 categories and can be performed on most of the general population.

48. A: A thorough comprehensive assessment (to include physical and mental evaluation) is imperative in order to place a patient into an appropriate therapeutic recreation program. It is important to assess the patient's level of functioning, along with learning their interests and cognitive level, in order for them to gain the most value of their recreation program. Their physical, as well as mental, health need to also be considered in order for the program to be effective.

49. C: Problem solving skills would be part of a cognitive assessment. The other elements listed are part of the affective assessment that is performed by the Recreation Therapist. Feelings of self-worth, facial expressions, and nonverbal body cues can all give information as to the patient's ability and willingness to participate in a therapeutic recreational therapy program.

50. D: The Leisure Diagnostic Battery, or LDB, measures current level of leisure functioning, along with measuring their perceived freedom in leisure activities. It consists of five sections: perception of freedom in leisure, perceived leisure control, leisure needs, depth of involvement, and playfulness. This tool can help to identify areas that are in need of improvement that impact leisure activities.

51. B: The physical assessment is the portion of the assessment that includes evaluation of a patient's ability to perform recreation activities. This includes evaluating motor skills and fitness level. Accurately assessing these components of a patient's abilities helps to place them in appropriate recreation and leisure activities that are appropriate for their functional level.

52. C: The Free Time Boredom Assessment identifies the component of free time that needs to be addressed. This can include physical involvement, mental involvement, meaningfulness, and speed of time. These areas are identified to avoid free time leading to boredom which can lead to poor choices regarding activities.

53. B: A 2009 study reported that 52% of physical therapists responding did not use standardized assessment tools. Of these, 49% did not plan to use standardized testing in the future. A 2011 study found that only 5% of RTs used the most common commercially available standardized tests like CERT, FOX, REDS, LCM, LDB, or Leisurescope, rather than 50% (A). Moreover, of the RTs responding in this study, a total of only 20% used any commercial standardized assessments. Some 2003 research found that mental health professionals tended to monitor patient/client progress more by using their own intuition than standardized instruments (C). Therefore, TR is NOT unique among therapeutic fields for its practitioners' lack of using available standardized testing instruments (D).

54. D: The majority of practicing RTs currently are more likely to use their clinical judgment—i.e. what they think about a client's status, informed by their training and experience—than to use clinical evaluation—i.e., valuing client attributes relative to positively changing their status, informed by valid and reliable assessment processes and instruments. Since they tend to use one of these rather than the other, (A) and (B) are incorrect; and (C) identifies the one they tend not to use.

55. A: The Leisure Constraints Index (L-CON) of the LAI assesses the extent of internal and external factors that restrict a person's participation in leisure activities and how much the person's perceived freedom is limited in the area of leisure. The LAP (B) assesses a person's repertoire of and involvement in various leisure activities. The L-PREF (C) assesses a person's preference among leisure activities, in which activities the person is interested in increasing participation; and the person's amount of self-determination in leisure through measuring his or her continuing involvement in activities s/he prefers. The L-INT (D) assesses which activities a person is interested in participating in but has unmet needs in by not participating in them or being unable to participate.

56. D: The validity of an assessment instrument means statistically that it measures what it intends and professes to measure. If an assessment instrument produces stable results when reused over time (A), this is the statistical definition of reliability rather than of validity. Validity does not mean both of these (B). (C) is a restatement of the concept behind reliability rather than validity.

57. A: This description refers to content validity, i.e. whether a test represents all of the content of the construct or behavior being measured. Construct validity (B) refers to how much a test measures the hypothetical construct it is meant to measure. Convergent validity (C) refers to how much a test's scores correlate with scores on other tests designed to measure the same construct (e.g. math ability). Discriminant validity (D) refers to how much a test's scores differ from the scores of tests that measure a different construct (e.g. math ability vs. verbal ability).

58. B: Concurrent validity refers to the extent that a test's scores correlate with the scores on another, similar, established test when both are administered at the same time (= concurrently). Predictive validity (A) follows the same logic; however, it refers to the extent that a test's scores will predict the same test's future scores when administered at two different times. Construct validity (C) refers to the extent to which a test measures the mental construct it is intended to measure (e.g. intelligence or creativity). Content validity (D) refers to the extent to which a test covers all of the content contained within the mental construct it is meant to measure.

59. B: Test-retest reliability (A), alternate-forms or equivalent-forms reliability (C), and split-half reliability (D) are all types of reliability that are determined by computing a correlation coefficient.

60. A: A constant (or systematic) error of measurement is one that occurs consistently in a test instrument, rendering it less valid—i.e. less likely to measure what it intends and/or purports to measure. A random error (B) of measurement is one that occurs randomly (not predictably or consistently), rendering a test instrument less reliable—i.e. less likely to yield consistent or stable scores over time and repeated administrations. Therefore, both (C) and (D) are incorrect.

61. D: Split-half reliability can be established through only one test administration, by dividing a test (especially a long test) in two by separating odd from even item numbers to produce two shorter tests. (This requires applying a correction formula, e.g. the Spearman-Brown prophecy formula, to the correlation coefficient since the two shorter tests are only half the length of the original and longer tests have higher reliability.) Alternate-forms reliability (A) requires two administrations, one for each of two different forms of the same test. Test-retest reliability (B) requires two administrations, one for the first testing and another for the retesting, to compare their results. Therefore, (C) is incorrect.

62. C: This relates to the purpose of the assessment. If the client is permanently physically unable to participate in some activities, the RT should give the client an assessment of leisure abilities. Assessing leisure interests is also important to a comprehensive evaluation, but it will not determine in which activities the client can actually participate. Availability (A) refers to whether the RT can obtain and administer a given assessment or not. Validity (B) refers to whether a given assessment tests what it is supposed to test. Reliability (D) refers to whether a given assessment produces consistent results across repeated administrations.

63. A: The first step in implementing assessment is to review the test protocol. The second step is to prepare for the assessment; the third is to administer the assessment. The fourth step is scoring and/or analyzing the results of the assessment. The fifth step is interpreting the results or score(s). The sixth step is documenting the results and interpretation of the assessment. The seventh step is reassessing the client as needed.

64. A: Structured interviews commonly involve standardized interview scripts, and the interviewer gives the respondent a choice of answers from which to select. Unstructured (B) interviews have no prewritten script, are more similar to conversations, and are more likely to involve more open-ended questions to which the respondent chooses his/her own answers. Semi-structured (C) interviews typically use questions that are both prewritten and also open-ended in nature, and the interviewer follows up the respondent's answers with probes to elicit additional information. Therefore, (D) is incorrect.

65. B: Assessment of the things described involves the Sensory functional domain. Assessment of the Cognitive (A) functional domain involves things like short-term and long-term memory; alertness and orientation; safety awareness; problem-solving ability; attention span, etc. Assessment of the Physical (C) functional domain involves things like general physical fitness; gross motor skills; fine motor skills; eye-hand coordination, etc. Assessment of the Social (D) functional domain involves things like interpersonal interactions; ability to form and sustain friendships; communication skills, including the ability to start and continue conversations and the ability to answer questions appropriately; ability to develop support networks, etc.

66. C: Assessment of leisure constraints is synonymous with assessment of leisure barriers. Both mean assessment of what factors interfere with a person's participation in leisure activities. Assessment of leisure skills (A) relates to assessing what knowledge and abilities a person has for various leisure activities. Assessment of leisure values (B) relates to assessing which kinds of leisure activities a person appreciates and does not appreciate. Assessment of leisure interests (D) relates to assessing which kinds of leisure activities a person most enjoys participating in most; and/or which activities s/he does not participate in but wants to, or wants to participate in more than s/he currently does.

67. B: The WHODAS 2,0 is a self-administered assessment used to assess the level of health and disability an individual is experiencing. It has proven reliable across cultures and can be used by the recreational therapist at the onset of therapy and to measure progress of therapeutic interventions. The World Health Organization emphasizes the use of this tool across health professions both in the setting of mental health and physical health and well-being.

68. B: Not allowing the diabetic patient with loss of sensation to sit for long periods of time without making sure that pressure is released shows that the RT anticipates a contraindication based on the patient's diagnosis. Loss of sensation secondary to diabetes is caused by circulatory inadequacy, and prolonged pressure that the patient cannot feel can lead to tissue damage. (A) is incorrect because an important recommendation for diabetics is to get regular exercise. (C) is incorrect because diabetics are advised to eat regularly, and especially before and/or after exercise, to maintain stable blood sugar levels. (D) is incorrect because a normal blood sugar check is an indication that exercise is acceptable. If the patient's blood sugar tested high or low, then exercise should be deferred until it has been normalized with insulin or food.

69. B: The RT should be aware that all these and more can be side-effects of seizure medications. All seizure medications can cause confusion (A), dizziness and lack of coordination (C); and some (e.g. Klonopin/Clonazepam) can cause low blood pressure, decreased respiration, and heart arrhythmias (D). These symptoms can all have significant impacts on physical activities, as well as on mental forms of recreation.

70. D: The RT can use the intake assessment report on a patient to make sure the TR goals s/he sets for the patient are consistent with the treatment goals set by the patient's lead doctor. The intake assessment report can be made by *any* approved professional whose duties include developing the care plan for the patient, not only by a certain professional (A). In community settings, the TR assessment will be the primary assessment; there will typically not be a prescription from a doctor (B). Using the information in the intake assessment report *will* help the RT to identify suitable topics and questions for further interviewing the patient (C).

71. B: The most objective way to provide concrete evidence of patient progress is by comparing current measures of patient performance to the same measures taken as baselines levels before the patient began treatment. While the RT's intuition (A), the agreement of all members on the treatment team that the patient has progressed (C), and the patient's self-report of his/her own experience of improvement (D) are valuable and may be accurate, they are also more subjective than quantitative measures of current performance that consistently exceed measures of baseline performance levels.

72. B: The Annual/Change of Condition/Re-Admit Assessment helps RTs to monitor and track changes in resident levels of functioning, which change individual resident needs, and adjust the TR program accordingly with those changes. The Intake Assessment (A) measures initial levels of functioning rather than subsequent changes in functioning levels. The Care Plan Section (C) helps RTs to write goals for the resident's care plan rather than monitoring changes in functioning levels. The Progress Note Section (D) helps TR professionals assess resident progress toward meeting the goals in their care plans and also evaluate the effectiveness of the plan rather than monitor changes in resident functioning levels.

73. A: Inclusive recreation enables people with disabilities to participate in the same activities that are offered to people without disabilities, e.g. children in schools and adults in their communities. TR/RT as a treatment modality (B) uses TR/RT to treat a diagnosed illness or condition, but does not require inclusion. TR/RT as a recreative process (C) introduces participants to different experiences of recreation and stresses that everyone has a right to recreation, but does not require inclusion. TR/RT from a holistic approach (D) addresses the individual as a whole person including all of his/her needs rather than focusing only on treating a problem, but does not require inclusion.

74. C: The Leisure Ability model of TR/RT is a continuum, moving from maximum control by the therapist to minimum control as the patient/client gains skills until s/he voluntarily participates. It includes four steps: assessment, treatment, leisure education, and leisure lifestyle. The Health Protection/Health Promotion model (A) is a treatment or medical model that focuses on treatment or rehabilitation for restoring health as health protection, and wellness-oriented activity for maintaining and/or enhancing optimal health as health promotion. It has three major components: prescriptive activities, recreation, and leisure. The TR Service Delivery model (B) establishes a framework for TR practice by helping practitioners to choose, organize, and sequence the services and interventions they provide. It has four components (diagnosis/needs assessment, treatment/rehabilitation, educational services, and prevention/health promotion; however, it focuses more on an overview of service delivery than on a continuum. The Ecological model (D) focuses on the environment and what in it must be changed, with changes including both eliminating personal barriers and promoting personal abilities.

75. C: The Health Protection/Health Promotion model (Austin, 1991) of TR/RT is theoretically based on humanistic psychology, which emphasizes the actualizing tendency to realize one's fullest potentials. In terms of protecting and promoting health, this self-actualization takes the form of achieving optimal wellness. Learned helplessness (A), intrinsic motivation (B), and locus of control (D) are all psychology concepts more closely associated with the Leisure Ability model of TR/RT.

76. A: Recreational therapists practice in a wide range of settings—not only in hospitals, rehabilitation facilities and nursing homes, etc., but also in private and public school systems (B), psychiatric facilities (C), and in clients' homes (D) as private practitioners and/or employees of home health care agencies.

77. D: ATRA Standard 9, Staff Qualifications and Competency Assessment includes the provision by TR Departments of professional development opportunities for its employees, as well as ensuring they hold the proper credentials. Standard 10, Quality Management (A), includes a TR Department's having a systematic, objective program that monitors and evaluates the appropriateness and quality of care and identifies and solves problems for improving TR services. Standard 8, Written Plan of Operation (B) requires TR Departments to operate according to a written plan of operation based on the ATRA Standards, and on other agencies' standards as indicated. Standard 12, Program Evaluation and Research (C) stipulates systematic and routine program evaluation and research by TR Departments for ascertaining how effective and suitable their programs are.

78. D: Principle 7, Informed Consent, in the ATRA Code of Ethics states that RTs are responsible to provide enough information about services, benefits, results, treatment duration, activities proposed, limitations, risks, and the credentials and training of the RT to prospective patients/clients that they are able to make a "reasoned decision" whether to accept or decline treatment. Principle 1, Beneficence (A), states that RTs will treat those they serve ethically by striving to maximize the potential benefits of treatment and minimize any potential harm. Principle 9, Competence (B) states that RTs are responsible for retaining and enhancing their own professional knowledge and credentials, and to deep their practices competent and current. Principle 8, Confidentiality (C) and Privacy, states that it is the duty of RTs not to give private information to third parties, and to inform patients/clients if such disclosure is required.

79. B: Canceling appointments *very frequently* (not just sometimes if unavoidable) could violate the ATRA Code of Ethics Principle 5, Fidelity, which states that RTs are obligated "to be loyal, faithful, and meet commitments made to persons receiving services." It could not violate ATRA Code of Ethics Principle 6, Veracity (A), which states that RTs "shall be truthful and honest" and avoid deception. While this behavior may reflect time management and/or other issues, it *does* violate an ethical principle, so (C) is incorrect. ATRA Code of Ethics Principle 2, Non-Maleficence, states the obligation of RTs to protect people from harm; this behavior could possibly violate this principle *indirectly* by not providing services as scheduled, but it does not *directly* violate it (D) as much as it would violate the Fidelity principle by not meeting commitments made to people who receive the RT's services.

80. B: Endurance reflects the individual's capacity for withstanding physical exertion over durations of time. Balance (A) reflects the person's ability to maintain body positions without toppling over and to right his or her body as needed. Activity level (C) reflects the relative intensity of the person's sensory system and body movements. Coordination (D) reflects how well the person's sensory system and body parts work together.

81. A: According to TR experts, strength includes not only a person's capacity for physical exertion and bearing weight, but also for flexibility in stretching and bending. Wellness (B) is more closely associated with a person's overall state of physical health. Endurance (C) relates to a person's ability to withstand physical exertion over time. Coordination (D) is more closely associated with how well a person's body parts and sensory system function in concert with each other.

82. B: Experts in the field note that although it is impossible to measure whether and how much a client is improving without first establishing a baseline of the client's behaviors using standardized assessment instruments, this does not happen most of the time. For example, recent (2011) research finds 96% of RTs screen client leisure history and interests using *non*-standardized interviews (A). Another issue is that the majority of RTs do NOT have adequate education about standardized assessment instruments that are appropriate, relevant, and apply to their RT practice (C). It is more common for most RTs NOT to employ standardized tools to measure specific areas of client functioning and/or treatments that target specific areas (D).

83. C: The ATRA's Standards for Practice include Standard 1, stating that TR specialists conduct assessments that are individualized, systematic, comprehensive, and accurate for deciding which course of action to take and what individualized treatment to plan for each client. They also include Standard 4, stating that TR specialists use systematic evaluations to assess client response to the treatment plan, i.e. to monitor client progress and treatment effectiveness; and to change the treatment plan as needed. Additionally, Standard 12 dictates "routine, systematic program evaluation and research for the purpose of determining appropriateness and efficacy." Thus, there are three ATRA standards of practice relating to assessment in some way; therefore, (A), (B), and (D) are incorrect.

84. C: The Comprehensive Assessment in Recreational Therapy (CERT)-Physical Disabilities is used to test a person's functional abilities in gross motor function, fine motor function, locomotion, motor skills, sensory function, cognition, communication, and behavior relative to leisure skills. The Idyll Arbor Leisure Battery (A) includes four subscales to measure leisure attitude, leisure interest, leisure motivation, and leisure satisfaction; none of these is used to assess physical functional skills. The FOX Activity Therapy Skills Baseline (B) is used to assess client skills in the social and affective domains rather than functional skills in the physical domain. The CERT-PSYCH-R (D) or Comprehensive Assessment in Recreational Therapy-Revised is used to assess a client's skills in social interaction rather than functional skills.

85. B: None of these is true about the TRAA (Hoss, 1993): It measures gross motor skills, fine motor skills, and also measures social behaviors (A) as well as communication skills (C) and cognitive skills (D).

86. A: The definition of an instrument's statistical reliability is that it can be repeated and yield stable results over time. This does not mean it is valid (B); the definition of statistical validity is that the instrument measures what it means and claims to measure. An instrument can be reliable without necessarily being valid, and the definitions of the two are not the same (C). The description given fits the definition of reliability, so its meaning neither (D) is incorrect.

87. D: Construct validity refers to how well a test measures the abstract/hypothetical idea or construct it is intended to measure. How well a test represents the entire subject, behavior, or construct it tests (A) is a definition of content validity, i.e. how well the test represents all of that subject's content. How well a test's current scores show what its future scores will be (B) is a definition of predictive validity (i.e. how well the current administration's scores predict a future administration's scores), also called criterion-related validity. How well a test's scores relate to a similar test's scores when they are given at the same time (C) is a definition of concurrent validity.

88. C: Construct validity is how much a test measures the abstract or hypothetical construct it is meant to measure. This can be obtained through experimentation and/or statistical correlation using a correlation coefficient (e.g. Pearson product-moment correlation, rank correlation, Cronbach's alpha, etc.) Face validity (A) means that the test appears on the face of it to measure what it intends to measure; this does not involve statistical computation to determine exactly how much it does so. Criterion validity (B), or criterion-oriented validity, also called predictive validity, means how much the scores on a current administration of a given test can predict the scores on that same test when given in a future administration. Concurrent validity (D) means how much a test's scores correlate with the scores on another, similar test when both are administered at the same time.

89. C: Random errors of measurement affect the reliability of a test by making its results differ from one time to the next. This makes the results less consistent and stable across administrations, i.e. less reliable. Constant errors (A), aka systematic errors, are errors of measurement that affect the validity of a test rather than its reliability. They make the test less likely to measure what it means and/or claims to measure. Therefore (B) and (D) are incorrect.

90. B: Test-retest reliability assesses how reliable a certain test is by administering it to the same person(s) at two different times and comparing the scores from both administrations. An inherent problem with determining this type of reliability is that the same test-taker(s) can have matured and/or learned more between administrations, and/or may remember material from taking the test during the earlier administration. Inter-rater reliability (A) assesses how consistent a test's scores are when scored by different raters or scorers. Alternate-forms reliability (C), also called equivalent-forms reliability, assesses test consistency by administering two different forms of the same test: the tests are exactly the same in content, but the actual test items differ between the two. Internal consistency reliability (D) assesses how consistent all of a test's items are with one another.

91. A: Rationale equivalence reliability is NOT established by computing a correlation; rather, it estimates how internally consistent a test is by how well each of the test's items relates to all of the other items on that same test. Equivalent-forms reliability (B) is established by computing the correlation between different forms of the same test with identical content but different items. Test-retest reliability (C) is established by computing the correlation between the scores from one administration of a test and from a later administration of the same test. Split-half reliability (D) is established by computing the correlation between the scores from administrations of two different halves of the same test.

92. B: This relates to the criterion of practicality: it is not practical or realistic to give a long test requiring focused attention for lengthy periods of time to a child who is young and/or diagnosed with ADHD as the test's qualities will make it difficult or impossible for such a client to respond adequately. A test that can be administered in a short time (or given in short segments at different times), and that does not require as much attentional focus, would be more practical. Availability (A) relates to whether the RT can obtain and administer the chosen test or not. Reliability (C) relates to how stable or consistent the test's results have been determined to be over repeated administrations. Purpose (D) relates to why the test is selected; for example, one would not choose a test that assesses social skills to determine a client's motor skills, or vice versa.

93. C: How long the patient can attend to something, i.e. attention span, should be measured objectively and is part of the assessment of the cognitive domain of functioning, rather than of behavioral observations related to assessment. Behavioral observations can include observing the amount, frequency, and types of motor activity the patient demonstrates (A); observing the kind of body language the patient displays and what messages it conveys (B); and observing how the patient interacts with other people, 1:1 and in social situations (D).

94. B: The tests named are examples of functional assessments. Some examples of leisure assessments (A) include the Leisure Diagnostic Battery (LDB), Leisurescope Plus series, and the Leisure Competence Measure (LCM). Some examples of neurological assessments (C) include the

Rancho Los Amigos Scale; the Glasgow Coma Scale; and the Children's Coma Scale. Some examples of rehabilitation assessments (D) include the Functional Independence Measure (FIM); the Inpatient Rehabilitation Facility-Patient Assessment Inventory (IRF-PAI); and the American Spinal Association (ASIA) Scale.

95. B: Safety awareness and problem-solving ability belong in the Cognitive functional domain of the assessment. The Emotional (A) domain might involve assessing how the patient expresses feelings, whether s/he expresses anger in appropriate ways, and what the RT perceives the patient's attitude toward himself or herself to be. The Sensory (C) domain would involve assessing whether the patient can see and hear normally, feel tactile sensations normally (e.g. some diabetics have numbness or loss of sensation in their extremities), and/or is tactile-defensive (resists being touched). The Physical (D) domain would include assessing the patient's gross and fine motor skills, eye-hand coordination, general physical fitness, activities of daily living (ADLs), and other functional physical abilities.

96. C: In the four primary motivations for leisure activity identified by research, the motivator of stimulus avoidance is reflected by the degree to which a person engages in leisure activity to escape from life situations that are over-stimulating. Intellectual motivation (A) for leisure is reflected by the degree to which a person wants to participate in leisure activities involving mental processes like exploration, discovery, imagination, creation, and/or learning. Competence mastery (B) reflects the degree to which a person engages in leisure activities for the purposes of competing with self and/or others, achieving accomplishments, challenging self and/or others, and mastering skills. Social motivation (D) reflects the degree to which a person engages in leisure activities for the purposes of forming and/or maintaining interpersonal relationships and friendships, and of feeling valued by others.

97. C: The patient's medical charts would be the RT's best source of assessment data concerning how many times s/he has had surgery, as these operations must all be documented. The family history (A) is a better source of data about the patient's upbringing, current family members, etc. Family interviews (B) can often access more detailed information than doctors may have, but usually about other factors like the patient's past and current leisure activities and interests, social interactions, relationships, behaviors, health status outside of hospitalizations and doctor visits, etc. Other members of the treatment team (D) may not have any more information about the patient's surgeries than the RT does if none has previous knowledge of the patient; and regardless, the medical charts should give more complete records including exact dates of surgeries, complications, etc.

98. B: Research has found that while exercise rehabilitation does NOT make MS symptoms worse (A) and does NOT increase relapse rates for MS patients (C), neither does it actually reverse the progression of the neurological impairments caused by MS (D); however, it CAN benefit MS patients by improving their physical and neurological functioning and their quality of life.

99. B: The first thing the RT should consider when observing the symptoms described is that they are common side-effects of many seizure medications. Because the patient has a seizure disorder, the RT should not first assume the patient also has an alcohol or drug addiction (A) or a mental illness (C) because these symptoms are more likely to be due to medication to control the seizures. The symptoms described are not common side-effects of seizure disorders themselves (D), but do often occur as side-effects of anti-seizure medications.

100. B: When an assessment is a published, standardized instrument, the manufacturer has used either norm-referencing (i.e. the scores obtained by the user are compared to norms or average scores of a sample representative of the intended population) or criterion-referencing (i.e. the scores obtained are compared to some criteria that have been previously established). To interpret a patient's test scores accurately, the RT must do so as the test manufacturer meant them to be interpreted, using the norm-referencing or criterion-referencing specified. Since the manufacturer may have used either norms or criteria, (A) and (C) are incorrect. Since the manufacturer of a published, standardized assessment has used one or the other of these, (D) is incorrect.

101. A: The Measurement of Social Empowerment and Trust (SET) evaluates changes in a patient's social skills and social attitudes as results of treatment. The Leisure Satisfaction Measure (B) assesses how well a person feels his/her needs are met by leisure activity. This can help RTs evaluate whether existing leisure programs meet the person's needs and which kinds of TR interventions can improve the person's leisure satisfaction; but other than regarding leisure satisfaction, it would not inform as much about progress in social skills, leisure skills, or other aspects of treatment progress. The Leisure Interest Measure (C) identifies relative interest for activities in each of eight leisure activity domains. This informative to RTs for providing activities of interest to patients, and educating patients to promote interest in more domains, but less for assessing treatment progress. The Leisure Motivation Scale (D) assesses what areas (intellectual, social, competence-mastery, and/or stimulus-avoidance) motivate an individual to engage in leisure activities rather than treatment progress.

102. A: When a long-term care resident's needs change due to changes in levels of functioning, the Annual/Change of Condition/Re-Admit Assessment section will help the RT measure those changes and adjust the resident's individualized care plan accordingly. To evaluate a resident's initial functioning levels relative to recreation (B), the RT can use the Intake Assessment section of the MARRCC 2. To evaluate the resident's progress toward attaining the goals in his/her individualized care plan (C), and/or to assess the effectiveness of the individualized care plan (D), the RT can use the Progress Notes section of the MARRCC 2.

103. D: A sentinel event is defined by The Joint Commission as any event that occurs in a healthcare setting that results in the death or significant psychological damage of a patient. A root cause analysis is performed when a sentinel event takes place to identify the cause of the incident, as well as put forth measures to help prevent this from happening again.

104. B: SMART goals is an acronym for Specific, Measurable, Attainable, Relevant, and Timely. It assists in establishing specific objectives to be reached in order to accomplish a specific goal that has been identified. The SMART goals tool helps to identify the large, overall goal and assists in establishing smaller, intermediary goals that are achievable on the path toward achieving the main goal.

105. A: The FIM tool is most useful for documentation at the inpatient level. The acronym stands for Functional Independence Measure. This tool is used to evaluate the physical and cognitive progress of the patient undergoing different forms of rehabilitation. The cognitive portion of the assessment may not be appropriate for patients who have sustained spinal cord injuries. The physical evaluation is particularly helpful for the Recreation Therapist when evaluating response to a plan that has been put in place for a patient.

106. D: Any subjective information is documented in the "S" portion of a SOAP note. This would be any information given to the therapist by the patient. This can be documented in a direct quote. It should include any additional details that patient will share about they are feeling physically and mentally. The other components of the SOAP note are the Objective information gathered by the therapist, the Assessment to document a diagnosis, and the Plan to formulate an individualized care plan for the patient.

107. C: In the SOAP method, the RT would note which activities to use with a patient in the P or Plan part, which is also where the doctor would note which medications s/he is prescribing. The doctor would note the patient's diagnosis (A) in the A or Assessment part. Prior treatments and/or providers (B) would be noted in the S or Subjective part, along with the rest of a narrative describing the patient's presenting problem. This S or Subjective part is also where the patient's rating (commonly on a scale of 1-10) of how severe his/her pain is (D) would be noted.

108. A: The date of onset of an injury and the way that it occurred would be entered in the "S" or Subjective section of SOAP notes. This section also includes the chronology of the problem (i.e. whether it is constant, or varies, or occurs in episodes; whether it is worse or better since it began, etc.); quality and severity of pain; factors that make it better or worse; other symptoms; and other providers and treatments involved. The "O" or Objective section (B) includes factual measurements like vital signs, physical examination results, laboratory test values; age, height, weight, etc. The "A" or Assessment (C) section includes physicians' notes of medical diagnoses they made, and conclusions of the health care team members based on the patient data they have reviewed. The "P" or Plan section (D) includes notes by all involved healthcare professionals of what treatments they plan for the patient.

109. B: The FIM contains a total of 18 items. When the National Task Force of rehabilitation research was developing the FIM, its members reviewed 36 (A) scales of functional assessment, published and unpublished, in order to select the best instrument; but this number is not the number of items contained in the FIM. The FIM is an ordinal scale comprised of seven (C) levels; however, it includes a total of 18 items across these levels. It takes about 20 to 30 (D) minutes to complete the FIM; but this is not the number of items that it contains.

110. D: The FIM is designed to have sensitivity to changes in individual patients during the process of comprehensive medical rehab programs in inpatient settings. It has been found statistically to be both reliable (A) and valid (B). However, it is limited in its ability to evaluate patients with traumatic brain injuries due to a scarcity of functional items related to TBIs; hence it is not diagnosis-specific for assessing TBI survivors (C).

111. A: According to the Center for Outcome Measurement in Brain Injury (COMBI), the FIM is designed for evaluating areas of activity dysfunction typically experienced by people who have neurological, musculoskeletal, and other disorders that are either reversible, fixed (permanent), or progressive in nature. As the FIM instrument includes all of these types of disorders, none of them is an exception; hence (B), (C), and (D) are incorrect.

112. B: This is the best example because it includes the conditions (when asked or on request, and using the technique as taught); and an action verb indicating the desired performance (will climb). (A) is less specific and is a better example of a goal or an "enabling objective", which a more specific performance objective or measure could accompany. (C) is not as good because it says the client "will know" rather than using an active verb like "will climb": it is not possible to measure or quantify what the client knows without the client's demonstrating that knowledge by doing something. Similarly, (D) uses the unquantifiable, non-specific verb "understand" instead of "will climb".

113. D: The 2021 US Census found that the leisure activity that achieved the most hours per day by both sexes was watching TV, followed by socializing/communicating, then playing games and using the computer. This data is relevant to the nature of leisure activities most commonly practiced in the context of healthy habits and exercise.

114. B: Building a birdhouse is a good example of an appropriate choice of RT activity for addressing a client goal of following sequential instructions because it is an activity performed in steps taken in a certain order. Playing tag (A) is less appropriate for this goal because the game does not involve sequential steps as birdhouse building does. However, building a birdhouse is not as appropriate an activity choice to meet a client goal of improving socialization skills (C) because it is an activity the client can do alone without social interaction. Playing basketball is also less appropriate for a goal of improving social skills (D) than, for example, playing Bingo.

115. B: The hand-over-hand technique is most appropriate for doing crafts, a manual activity, with a client who has motor apraxia, which makes it difficult to direct and control one's physical movements. Reality therapy (A) is a type of psychotherapy for clients with psychiatric, psychological, emotional, and/or behavior disorders rather than for facilitating motor control. Sequencing steps (C) is a technique appropriate for clients who have difficulties with executive function, specifically cognitive processes that enable performing steps of a task in the correct order. Cognitive reframing (D) is a technique used in psychotherapy, particularly cognitive-behavioral therapy, to help a client view or approach an issue or situation in a different way.

116. B: Assistive computer technology allows persons with disabilities, including those with upper-body limitations, to write poetry, fiction, non-fiction, etc. People in wheelchairs can read books (A) without such technology; they may need adapted book holders, some of which also include page-turning capabilities. Most movie theatres today have seating areas with wheelchair access since the Americans with Disabilities Act (ADA) was passed in 1990, and wheelchair-bound disabled persons can go to the movies (C) without assistive computer technology. According to experts, watching TV (D) is the recreational activity most common to spinal cord injury patients. Spinal cord medicine authorities advise also encouraging activities that involve more active participation for these patients, but their watching TV does not require assistive computer technology.

117. A: Studies have shown that residents of long-term care facilities tend to show more objective signs of agitation when they are not occupied with an independent or social activity. This agitation can express itself in wandering behaviors, calling out, or even aggression. It has been found that occupying residents with an independent recreational activity, such as a craft project or a puzzle, can decrease these signs of agitation and help them to remain calm and less troubled.

118. C: Support groups allow a person to feel like they are not alone in their situation. They are a resource where someone can find ways to work through a specific problem or disability by learning from others who gone through the same process. A person is not required to speak and tell their own story, but it is often helpful to do so. The support group provides an opportunity to gain insight into a problem and learn how others have succeeded in adapting to that problem. Support group meetings should not be complaining or blaming sessions, but rather, a therapeutic environment for people to share, learn, and gain comfort.

119. C: Systematic desensitization gradually reduces fear/avoidance of stimuli through successive approximations (i.e. small steps) toward the dreaded stimulus. In agoraphobia, going out is the dreaded stimulus. The client receives training involving small steps until comfortable with each; e.g. first stepping out the apartment door; then walking down the hall; then getting on the elevator; then crossing the lobby; then stepping outside the building door; then taking a few steps down the sidewalk, etc. DRI (A) is often used to replace an unwanted behavior by reinforcing a desired behavior only when the undesired one does not occur; for example, reinforcing sitting but not running, or vice versa. DRO (B) reinforces a replacement behavior that is not necessarily incompatible, but different from the undesired behavior as long as the undesired behavior does not occur. Positive reinforcement (D), i.e. rewarding a desired behavior to increase its recurrence, is more powerful than punishing undesired behaviors, but alone is not as effective for agoraphobia as systematic desensitization.

120. A: Leisure counseling involves using a patient's past, present, and/or future recreational interests and activities for psychotherapeutic ends. Therapeutic domains that researchers have identified for the application of leisure counseling include alleviating the symptoms of phobias, panic attacks, and post-traumatic stress disorder (B); controlling and inhibiting obsessive, compulsive, and addictive behaviors (C); and aiding in the establishment and maintenance of positive moods (D).

121. D: In order to advocate for all kinds of people in delivering TR services, RTs should include activities in the programs they plan that cause the RTs, their clients, and everyone else involved to examine their own and others' biases (A), i.e. partiality against and/or for some kinds of people; phobias (B), i.e. exaggerated fears and/or aversions to some kinds of people; and prejudices (C), i.e. prejudgments or preconceived opinions about some kinds of people with no basis in fact, experience, or reasoning. This is a basic precept in TR/RT and in a democratic society. While examining disease etiology is an element of the RTs foundational knowledge, this is not as relevant when it comes to the nature and diversity of recreation and leisure activities for all kinds of people.

122. B: The Smart Glove is a technological assistive device that is worn by a patient during rehabilitation from a stroke or other condition that has affected their ability to achieve hand and finger mobility. It is operated through a Bluetooth connection to record the range of motion a person has while performing specific tasks, usually in a game format. The tasks can be individualized based on a patient's progress with achieving basic range of motion activities up to more advanced fine motor skills.

123. C: Independent ADLs are those activities of daily living that are not essential to providing basic hygiene or self-care. They add quality to life, but are not essential for daily living. These include housekeeping, shopping, managing money, and managing medications. Limitations with independent ADLs may come from a physical deficit that prevents a person from performing them, or a cognitive deficit that makes it difficult for them to follow the steps or understand these activities.

124. D: A vocational rehabilitation counselor assists people with disabilities in finding secure employment. This may often involve coordinating training for a new vocation or working with occupational and physical therapists to find adaptive techniques for someone to perform job duties. Employment can help to boost self-esteem and decrease depression or anxiety symptoms for those who are adjusting to a new physical disability.

125. A: The referring provider should be open with the patient regarding the need for a specialty consultation. The reason for the consultation, along with the names of appropriate providers should be discussed. Once the patient is in agreement to be referred, all pertinent records should be sent to the consultant so that he or she is adequately informed of the patient's history.

126. A: Having a patient with a hearing impairment offers the opportunity to utilize different forms of teaching. Some of these patients may have some degree of hearing acuity left, but most have learned to adapt and read lips. It is important to be aware of any distracting background noises and to face the patient directly so that one's face and mouth are clearly visible. Remember not to turn away when talking or cover the mouth with the hand as that will make it difficult for the patient.

127. D: The Purpose of TR program design means Why the program is created – for what reason or purpose it hopes to accomplish. The Population of TR program design means Who – for whom the program is created, i.e. the group of patients/clients to be served. The Process of TR program means How – what knowledge and skills are to be taught and/or improved, and what techniques and activities will be used to accomplish this learning. The Setting of TR program design means Where – i.e. in what location and type of environment (inpatient, outpatient, community, school, daycare, group home, hospital, institution, etc.) the program will be implemented.

128. D: Recreation Therapy is not currently able to bill Medicare for telehealth services. There are currently no telehealth-specific CPT codes available for billing for these services. Rarely, some private insurance policies will cover telehealth Recreation Therapy services, but this is not a standard service covered and patients will need to contact their insurance company to inquire about coverage. Medicaid does reimburse for telehealth services and has since 2002, but not in all 50 states.

129. B: Experiential therapies are those therapies that use actions, movements, and activities to treat the patient rather than traditional "talk" therapies. Recreational therapy falls under this umbrella. This approach is especially useful with teenagers who require therapy for mental illness and/or behavior issues. This type of therapy has been proven to improve cognitive and motor function.

130. C: TR services are most likely to use the Assessment, Plan, Implementation, and Evaluation or APIE process for designing specific interventions and programs in the areas of health care services, where TR services are usually prescribed by a doctor or a treatment team; and leisure services, where after being discharged from health care, patients often refer themselves seeking community-based TR. In transition services {(A), (B)}, TR services may be included in an Individualized Transition Plan or ITP, which contains goals and objectives for the client to achieve after completing school. In education services {(B), (D)}, TR services may be included in an Individualized Education Plan or IEP, which contains goals and objectives for a student to meet while in school and/or in a specific school program(s).

131. D: In service delivery systems, axes are ways of defining opposite/alternative/different types or sectors of service providers. Hence, providers may be either public or private (A), e.g. public schools vs. private schools; or government-funded rehabilitation facilities vs. privately funded rehabilitation facilities, etc.; profit or nonprofit (B), e.g. for-profit substance abuse recovery programs vs. nonprofit SA recovery programs; and clinical or community (C), e.g. inpatient medical clinics vs. outpatient community service centers, etc. Health and human services (D) do not represent two ends of an axis in service delivery systems. Rather, health services and human services are themselves two types of service delivery systems, which are often combined in government departments as Departments of Health and Human Services.

132. D: One of the purposes of developing the PPS for health care service delivery was to focus on client-centered or recipient-centered provision of services. Another purpose in developing the PPS *was* to control the costs of health care by pre-setting service prices (A). An additional purpose *was* to assure the quality of the health care services provided (B). And the PPS was also developed for the purpose of making sure that Medicare recipients *do* have access to the same health care services as others (C).

133. B: The Problem-Oriented Medical Record (POMR) is organized around patient problems, dividing the record into four parts: the data base, the problem list, the initial plan, and the progress notes. The Source-Oriented Medical Record (SOMR) does not do this (A). Instead, the SOMR divides the record by each discipline that is a source of data, with separate sections of the chart for medical notes, nursing notes, TR notes, etc. The POMR does not do this (C). Therefore, the SOMR and POMR do not both include all of these (D).

134. D: Considerations for RTs when evaluating their TR programs include whether the population identified/targeted received benefits from participating in a program; the cost of implementing the program; and the ratio of those benefits to those costs. RTs should also consider whether good results can be attributed to the program rather than to other factors (A) as part of determining the program's effectiveness. They should consider not only the effectiveness of the program as a whole, but moreover which activities within the program were more or less effective and important (B). They should also consider whether their program has been implemented correctly: if it is not implemented as planned, then effectiveness cannot be attributed to the program's design or planning (or even to the program itself), and the source of positive outcomes is unknown (C).

135. C: Quality improvement is instrumental in improving the way healthcare services are provided, while continually measuring the effect those changes have on the health status of the patients served. This is often measured through patient satisfaction information, and is employed through initiatives and evidence based practices.

136. D: RT/TR departments and agencies (and others) should include utilization reviews in their written plans of operations. Utilization review focuses on *both* resources of a department or agency that are over-utilized (A) *and* those that are under-utilized (B), not only one or the other. Utilization review not only targets inefficiency to eliminate or reduce it, but also examines an agency's or department's effectiveness (C) in utilizing its resources.

137. B: The analysis (A) phase of TR program planning reveals client needs and helps planners develop their mission statement and program goals. The investigation phase involves examining operational units among the resources the RTs have available, which can become parts of the program implementation to fulfill parts of the mission statement and goals. The determination (C) phase is when the planners decide which of these investigated operational units they will actually select for inclusion in the program. The conceptualization (D) is the phase wherein planners develop their mission statement and comprehensive program goals. This occurs following the analysis and prior to the investigation and determination.

138. B: The NCTRC requires that to supervise internships, an agency RT must have been a CTRS for at least one year. At a university, the NCTRC requirement for intern supervision is just to be a CTRS, but not for one year (A). Internship supervisors at agencies are required by the NCTRC to be employed there full-time; i.e. at least 32 hours per week, not 25 (C). NCTRC requirements also include that the internship supervisor at an agency have 50% of his or her job duties in an established TR program, rather than only 25% (D).

139. C: A third-party payer is an organization that pays for the medical expenses of a person. This is usually a health insurance company such as Medicare, Medicaid, or private health insurance. The patient is the first-party payer who purchases the health insurance policy.

140. A: Medicare Part A covers the services available outside of a physician's office. This includes hospitalization, skilled nursing home care for the first 100 days after a 3-day hospital stay, hospice care, home care, and laboratory tests. Medicare Part B covers the care provided within the physician's office.

141. B: Medicare is a federal health insurance program, and Medicaid is a combined federal and state health insurance program. Medicare provides health insurance for people age 65 and older, and for people with end-stage kidney disease or other specific disabilities; Medicaid is not restricted to patients aged 65 or older, but is based on individual patient needs and qualifications which vary by state. Thus (A) is incorrect. Medicare Part A provides for hospital care and home health care services, but not outpatient services (C). It also provides for skilled nursing care and hospice services. Medicare Part B provides for outpatient services but not hospital care or home health care (D). It also provides for doctor services, emergency department visits, medical equipment, and supplemental medical insurance.

142. A: The operating budget, aka the revenue and expense budget, for a TR/RT facility identifies its expenses for daily operations as well as its revenues for a one-year period, not 3-5 years (C). The facility's capital expenditure budget, however, usually covers a period of 3-5 years, not one (B); and addresses long-term planning rather than everyday expenses (D).

143. B: The National Council for Therapeutic Recreation Certification (NCTRC) is independent of the National Therapeutic Recreation Society (NTRS) and the American Therapeutic Recreation Association (NTRA) to assure it better relationships with regulatory bodies like the Joint Commission and the Commission on Accreditation of Rehabilitation Facilities (CARF) by not appearing biased in favor of the profession; hence (A) is incorrect. The NCTRC provides certification to RTs, whereas the Joint Commission and the CARF provide accreditation to TR agencies; hence (C) is incorrect. The NCTRC credentials are certifications. Registration is being listed on official rosters by national, state, or professional, government or non-government groups, which carries less authority than certification. Examples include the National Voluntary Registration Plan for Hospital Recreation Personnel from the Council for the Advancement of Hospital Recreation; and the National Therapeutic Recreation Society (NTRS)' Voluntary Registration Plan. Licensure is even more stringent than certification and depends on state government legislation; hence (D) is incorrect.

144. B: RTs can earn CEUs, e.g. for recertification purposes, but no more than 25 credits from presenting and/or publishing. Attendance to webinars and teleconferences IS approved the same as in-person class attendance (A) for continuing education. RTs CAN also earn continuing education credits for their academic theses or dissertations (C). 1 educational contact hour of continuing education is equivalent to 1 credit; however, 1 contact hour and 1 credit are equivalent to 0.1 CEU, not 1 (D).

145. C: Although a general requirement of many states in the USA for practicing TR/RT is usually at least a Bachelor's degree, the specific requirements to practice vary from state to state. There are no Federal regulations uniformly governing TR requirements in all states (A). Licensure and certification are not required in every US state (B); only a few states currently require licensure, and not all states require certification (D).

146. A: By regularly making reports to agency administrators of the progress of TR clients, services, and programs, the RT professional can best promote the value of the TRS program. Evidence of the positive results of the program can prove its value. Publishing journal articles (B) advances scholarship in the field as well as the professional's individual competence, but will not promote the TRS program's value as well to those who decide whether it will continue to exist, expand, be funded, etc. and to what extent. Presentations to volunteers (C) promotes public relations for TR but does not promote the TRS program value to those with power over its existence. Participation in meetings of professional groups (D) supports the individual RT's competence, but does not demonstrate the TRS program's value to the administration.

147. B: According to research (cf. Skalko, 2013), although there are roughly 14,000 CTRSs in the country, fewer than 3,000 of them belong to ATRA, even though ATRA is the largest national organization for TRs in the country (A). This ATRA membership is also only 1/14 of the 42,000 members in the AOTA (C), the national professional organization for OTs (occupational therapists), a profession that commonly collaborates with RTs. The AOTA has two full-time lobbyists, whereas the ATRA has one part-time council and volunteers. Moreover, in addition to many more members, the AOTA has a political action committee (PAC) with $200,000 of funding; whereas the ATRA PAC has $0 in funds (D).

148. B: The NCTRC will only accept continuing education pursued by CTRSs for credits or CEUs if that education directly reflects the knowledge areas identified in the NCTRC Job Analysis Study. This is one way to ensure that the continuing education CTRSs pursue contributes to the advancement of the TR/RT profession as well as to the competence of the individual CTRS professional. This requirement means that the NCTRC will NOT grant CEUs or credits for every experience a CTRS completes (A) if it is not relevant to any of the NCTRC Job Analysis knowledge areas. The NCTRC does not offer its own CE courses (C). However, it does offer links on its website to other organizations that do provide CE courses, including organizations offering CE through home study courses and professional journal review; but the NCTRC itself does not offer these (D).

149. C: Providers must be very cognizant of the relationships they establish with patients and their families. It is easy to become "attached" to patients, but it is unprofessional and harmful to place oneself in a position in which the relationship has lost the boundary between provider and patient. The recreational therapist must always be wary of the relationships established with patients and continue to re-evaluate those boundaries so that they are able to provide the best care to the patient as possible.

150. B: It is important to be aware of the conversations occurring around oneself, especially in a public place. HIPAA regulations prohibit conversations in a public space regarding a patient. It would be appropriate to subtly remind co-workers of this if it occurs.

Practice Test #2

1. The CTRS is encouraging team members to use the STAR approach to client safety. The CTRS explains that the STAR approach begins by

a. safeguarding clients.
b. stopping to concentrate on tasks.
c. securing needed equipment/tools.
d. selecting appropriate tasks.

2. A client with a history of aggression begins swearing and pacing back and forth, shouting, "You can't make me stay here!" The MOST appropriate initial response is to

a. speak calmly and quietly to the client.
b. tell the client this behavior is inappropriate.
c. leave the room.
d. call security to restrain the client.

3. In evaluating research as part of the development of evidence-based practice guidelines, the four evaluative/trustworthiness criteria are (1) credibility, (2) dependability, (3) transferability, and (4)

a. controllability.
b. applicability.
c. accountability.
d. confirmability.

4. A client with multiple sclerosis tells the CTRS that she is upset that she can no longer continue her employment because her job is too physically demanding and is concerned about how she will support herself. Which of the following responses focuses on problem solving as a response to stress?

a. "What options have you considered for less physically demanding work?"
b. "You might be eligible for public assistance."
c. "I'm sure there is other work you can do."
d. "I can see how upsetting that is for you."

5. According to the Joint Commission, which of the following is generally acceptable as one of two required identifiers?

a. Place of birth
b. Date of birth
c. Place of employment
d. Verifying client's name from armband taped to bedside stand

6. When advising parents about age-appropriate exercise for a 4-year-old child about to be discharged from the hospital after treatment for diabetes, which of the following activities is MOST appropriate?

a. Dancing or skating
b. Bicycling
c. Team sports
d. Gymnastics

7. Using the average cost of a problem and the cost of intervention to demonstrate savings is a(n)

a. cost-benefit analysis.
b. efficacy study.
c. product evaluation.
d. cost-effective analysis.

8. Listed below are the 5 stages of substance abuse:

1. Regular use.
2. Dependence.
3. Problem use.
4. Experimentation.
5. Addiction.

Which of the following correctly orders these stages from first to last?

a. 1, 2, 3, 4, 5
b. 3, 4, 2, 1, 5
c. 4, 1, 3, 2, 5
d. 4, 3, 2, 1, 5

9. Which of the following characteristics indicates that a dog is likely well-suited to be a therapy dog?

a. Guards toys and food
b. Likes to lick people
c. Very enthusiastic and excited about meeting people
d. Remains confident in different environments

10. If, when utilizing the Plan-Do-Study-Act (PDSA) method of continuous quality improvement, study of the outcomes of a trial indicates that the solution that was instituted was not effective, the next step is to

a. return to the Plan step.
b. return to the Do step.
c. discontinue the process.
d. continue to the Act step.

11. When reviewing a number of articles as part of development of evidence-based practice guidelines, the first step to reading critically should be to

a. review the author's credentials.
b. consider the source.
c. read the article conclusion.
d. evaluate the overall article.

12. The three primary elements of motivational interviewing are

a. collaboration, evocation, and autonomy.
b. orientation, identification, and termination.
c. input, discussion, output.
d. identification of barriers, conflict resolution, and implementation.

13. When entering the room of a client who is deaf and facing away from the door, the CTRS should

a. approach from the direction the client is facing.
b. say the client's name.
c. approach and touch the client.
d. clap hands or tap the foot.

14. If an adverse incident occurs, a written report should be completed

a. within 24 hours.
b. only if an injury occurred.
c. immediately or as soon as possible.
d. after discussion with risk management.

15. Which of the following poses the greatest barrier to communication?

a. The client is extremely anxious and crying.
b. The client is deaf and uses a sign-language interpreter.
c. The client is vision-impaired but sees shapes.
d. The client has mild cognitive impairment.

16. The best method of ensuring that a client follows the plan of care is to

a. write out directions clearly.
b. include the client in the planning.
c. ask a family member to supervise.
d. provide incentives.

17. The CTRS has called a client who is being treated for chronic depression because the client has missed one appointment and two sessions of the support group. The statement by the client that is of MOST concern is

a. "I don't like the support team leader, so I don't feel comfortable."
b. "I've been giving all my things away, and I feel so much better."
c. "I know that I need to keep my appointments, and I'll do better."
d. "My partner will be upset with me for not going to therapy."

18. If a stroke client has been discharged home but is having difficulty preparing foods because of residual right-sided weakness, the MOST appropriate referral is to a(n)

a. occupational therapist.
b. physical therapist.
c. home health aide.
d. meals-on-wheels program.

19. Which of the following is a nonverbal clue that a client may be anxious?

a. Client rubs his eyes and yawns
b. Client has flat affect and responds in monosyllables
c. Client's pupils are constricted and client sniffs repeatedly
d. Client rubs hands together constantly

20. When the CTRS is assisting a nonambulatory client to transfer from a wheelchair into an automobile, the BEST assistive device is likely a

a. lateral transfer device.
b. slip sheet.
c. sliding board.
d. transfer/pivot disc.

21. If a CTRS dislikes working with older adults and frequently avoids older clients while showing favoritism to young adults of a similar age to the CTRS, this is an example of

a. negligence.
b. incompetence.
c. boundary violation.
d. personal preference.

22. When interviewing a client whose culture is different from the CTRS, the CTRS asks what the client believes is the cause of the client's symptoms and what treatment the client expects. This is an example of

a. cultural competence.
b. insecurity.
c. motivational interviewing.
d. empowering.

23. The primary purpose of conducting a problem-based assessment of a client is to

a. focus on one problem.
b. review one body system.
c. focus on client history.
d. create a problem list.

24. Considering Tuckman's stages of group development, during which stage does the leader's input and direction decrease?

a. Forming.
b. Storming.
c. Norming.
d. Performing.

25. The four components of the Therapeutic Service Delivery Model (Van Andel) include (1) Diagnosis/Needs assessment, (2) Treatment/Rehabilitation, (3) Education, and (4)

a. Prevention/Health Promotion.
b. Self-determination.
c. Intrinsic/Extrinsic motivation.
d. Leisure lifestyle.

26. The primary goals of client advocacy are

a. providing direct services for clients.
b. lobbying administrative/legislative bodies for improved services.
c. increasing resources to better meet client needs.
d. promoting client independence and improvement in the healthcare system.

27. A client who is post-amputation of a lower limb and insists he needs no rehabilitation therapy is probably experiencing

a. self-confidence.
b. denial.
c. delusions.
d. fear.

28. The primary goal of rehabilitation for a client who has suffered a spinal cord injury is

a. promote independence.
b. promote psychological wellbeing.
c. prevent complications.
d. educate regarding rights of the disabled.

29. The type of managed care plan that allows a client to see physicians and care providers within a network but to seek outside treatment in some circumstances is

a. Health maintenance organization (HMO).
b. Exclusive provider organization (EPO).
c. Point of service plan (POS).
d. Preferred provider organization (PPO).

30. A bipolar client who is very nervous about transitioning into the community from a sheltered environment may benefit from

a. a support group.
b. a 12-step program.
c. an adult daycare program.
d. peer counseling.

31. When a client is receiving recreational therapy in the home, documentation must include

a. costs.
b. client preferences.
c. realistic and measurable goals.
d. indirect supervision of unlicensed staff.

32. The coping mechanism that involves actively searching for a way to reduce stress and cope is

a. problem-solving.
b. avoidance.
c. physical activity.
d. spirituality.

33. If all shelters are full and an indigent uninsured client with mental health issues and planned discharge in 3 days is placed on a waiting list for a preferred shelter, the next action should be to

a. call daily to determine where the client is on the list.
b. place the client on a second waiting list.
c. plan transfer to a skilled nursing facility until shelter placement is possible.
d. refer the problem to Social Services.

34. Durable medical equipment (DME) classified as assistive devices include

a. electric beds.
b. handrails.
c. crutches.
d. apnea/sleep monitors.

35. A 6-year-old hospitalized child is drawing a picture of a boy in a bed crying, with large tears on the face falling onto the pillows. Which of the following is the MOST appropriate statement to elicit the child's feelings?

a. "Why is the little boy in your picture crying?"
b. "Is the little boy afraid to be in the hospital?"
c. "I see that the little boy in your picture is crying."
d. "Did something hurt the little boy?"

36. When a client's spouse asks for information about another client, the response that complies with the Health Insurance Portability and Accountability Act (HIPAA) is

a. "The law doesn't allow me to give out any information about clients in order to protect their privacy and safety."
b. "His wife is in the lounge. You can go ask her."
c. "Why are you asking?"
d. "He has bipolar disease, like your husband."

37. At which time of day are clients with cognitive impairment usually MOST sensitive to sensory overload?

a. Noon
b. Early AM
c. Late evening
d. Afternoon

38. According to Maslow's Hierarchy of Needs, which of the client's needs must be met FIRST?

a. Safety and Security
b. Physiological
c. Belonging and self-esteem
d. Self-actualization

39. The primary goals of using play therapeutically with children include all of the following EXCEPT

a. establishing contact with the child.
b. interpreting the child's behavior.
c. assessing family dynamics.
d. observing and collecting data.

40. When encouraging a 4-year-old child to engage in healthcare play as doctor or nurse, which of the following is the BEST "patient" for the child?

a. A sibling
b. A parent
c. A doll or stuffed animal
d. The CTRS

41. When assessing a client's level of interest in activities, which of the following information MOST essential?

a. Type of activity, past and recent past interest, current participation, and future interest
b. Type of activity, availability of activity resources
c. Type of activity, cost of activity, feasibility of participation
d. Type of activity, physical ability, and current interest

42. A 22-year-old male with a T2 spinal cord injury attends a football game, sitting in the shade in his wheelchair for 3 hours in 92° weather at 85% humidity. Which of the following is the PRIMARY concern?

a. Overheating
b. Dehydration
c. Pressure sore
d. Bladder distention

43. Which of the following is a central concept of Bandura's (1977, 2001) Social Learning Theory?

a. Stimulus-response
b. Information processing
c. Perception
d. Role modeling

44. Which of the following is the first step to conducting a program evaluation?

a. Determining the purpose
b. Selecting evaluators
c. Selecting an evaluation design
d. Identifying the time frame

45. If using the DARP focused charting format, DARP stands for

a. date, assessment, resource, prevention.
b. data, action, response, plan.
c. duration, assessment, reaction, participation.
d. discuss, act, respond, plan.

46. Which of the following is an appropriate activity for a client who needs low impact physical exercise?

a. Running in place
b. Playing tennis
c. Water aerobics
d. Bicycling

47. According to Kolb's Experiential Learning Theory, what type of learning style corresponds to a person who likes working with people?

a. Convergent
b. Assimilative
c. Accommodative
d. Divergent

48. Which of the following federal legislations/agencies require that parks and recreation facilities serve people with disabilities, including eliminating architectural barriers to access?

a. Occupational Safety and Health Administration
b. Americans with Disabilities Act
c. Health Insurance Portability and Accountability Act
d. Individuals with Disabilities Education Act

49. All of the following are assessed as part of the Instrumental Activities of Daily Living instrument EXCEPT

a. bathing.
b. food preparation.
c. housekeeping.
d. telephone use.

50. In order to receive accreditation from the Commission on Accreditation of Rehabilitation Facilities (CARF), the most important responsibility is to

a. pay annual fees to CARF.
b. avoid any conflicts of interest with other accreditation agencies.
c. establish standards based on local practice.
d. conform to internationally accepted standards.

51. The goal of the Leisure Ability Model of treatment is for the client to

a. rapidly achieve maximum mobility.
b. depend on the CTRS for guidance throughout treatment.
c. become increasingly independent in treatment/activities.
d. come to terms with disability.

52. Which of the following is a specialization area recognized by the NCTRC for certification?

a. Cultural competence
b. Adolescent health
c. Community inclusion services
d. Psychological services

53. Under the Individuals with Disabilities Education Act, therapeutic recreation is generally indicated as a

a. primary service.
b. related service.
c. non-covered service.
d. counseling service.

54. All of the following are characteristics of addictive personalities EXCEPT

a. approval-seeking.
b. impulsive.
c. thrill-seeking.
d. lying.

55. According to the Self-Determination Theory (Ryan and Deci), intrinsic motivation is diminished by

a. autonomy.
b. demonstration of competence.
c. encouragement.
d. external rewards.

56. A client who wants to play table tennis again after an injury has poor manual strength and limited dexterity. The best solution is likely

a. suggesting another activity.
b. playing a video simulation.
c. utilizing an adaptive glove.
d. using a larger paddle.

57. If the CTRS is applying for recertification under option 1, how many hours of work and continuing education are required?

a. 1200 hours of work and 30 hours of continuing education
b. 800 hours of work and 40 hours of continuing education
c. 480 hours work and 50 hours continuing education
d. 240 hours of work and 25 hours continuing education

58. Which of the following elements is an essential part of mentoring a novice CTRS?

a. Providing discipline
b. Providing feedback
c. Providing a formal evaluation
d. Providing criticism

59. According to Principle 9 (Competence) of the ATRA Code of Ethics, the CTRS is responsible for

a. continually seeking to expand knowledge in recreation therapy.
b. working toward advance degrees in recreation therapy.
c. mentoring and supervising other recreational therapists.
d. reporting violations of professional boundaries.

60. If the CTRS is interested in working with an intern in the field of recreation therapy, the best marketing method is likely to

a. send a letter/email to schools with recreation therapy programs.
b. contact other individual CTRSs.
c. post a notice in a recreational therapy journal.
d. wait until contacted by a university program.

61. Which of the following reviews the necessity of care in relation to admission, treatment, and discharge?

a. Risk management
b. Record review
c. Process variance monitoring
d. Utilization review

62. Listed below are the 4 steps of risk management.

1. analysis.
2. identification.
3. assessment.
4. prevention.

Which of the following correctly orders these steps from first to last?

a. 1, 2, 3, 4
b. 2, 1, 4, 3
c. 3, 2, 1, 4
d. 4, 1, 2, 3

63. The four elements of intervention that are of primary importance in the Therapeutic Recreation Accountability Model (TRAM) include

a. program design, client assessment, documentation, and program evaluation.
b. plan, assess, treat, review.
c. assessment implementation, treatment plans, progress notes, and discharge/referral summaries.
d. Protocol development, client assessment plan, program outcomes, and client outcomes.

64. If someone has made a verbal complaint about a grievance to the program director but believes the response was inadequate, the next step should be to

a. file a formal written complaint.
b. complain in person to the board of directors.
c. speak to the director again.
d. notify the state medical board.

65. Risk management includes determining the burden of proof for negligent acts. Which of the following types of negligence refers to willfully providing inadequate care without regard to the safety and security of the client?

a. Contributory negligence
b. Comparative negligence
c. Negligent conduct
d. Gross negligence

66. The primary advantage of just-in-time ordering of inventory is

a. time saving.
b. cost saving.
c. flexibility.
d. labor saving.

67. Which type of budget finances daily operations and includes general expenses, such as salaries?

a. Operating
b. Cash balance
c. Master
d. Capital

68. If a CTRS is to undergo peer review, the CTRS should expect that review will be carried out by

a. someone who works in the same unit/department.
b. a CTRS with similar work experience.
c. a team of staff members, including a CTRS.
d. a CTRS of the his/her choosing.

69. When supervising another staff member, the CTRS should focus on

a. what the person is doing correctly.
b. what the person is doing incorrectly.
c. areas for improvement.
d. educational needs.

70. Which of the following models/theories suggests that a client's health behavior is influenced by 8 beliefs, including perceived benefits, barriers, and the ability to overcome barriers?

a. Stress-coping model
b. Social learning theory
c. Self-determination model
d. Health Protection/Health Promotion Model

71. Listed below are the 5 steps to clinical problem solving:

1. Collect data.
2. Make decision.
3. Identify important concepts.
4. Define the issue.
5. Consider reasons for actions.

Which of the following correctly orders these steps from first to last?

a. 1, 4, 3, 5, 2
b. 5, 4, 3, 1, 2
c. 4, 1, 3, 5, 2
d. 3, 4, 5, 1, 2

72. Which of the following solutions is the MOST appropriate for a visually-impaired client who wants to participate in team sports, such as baseball?

a. Use a Beeper ball
b. Utilize adaptive gloves
c. Have a one-on-one coach
d. Hand out supplies to others

73. The primary purpose of palliative care is to

a. provide end-of-life care.
b. relieve pain and discomfort.
c. prevent progression of disease.
d. prevent complications.

74. Under the International Classification of Functioning (WHO), the performance qualifier for Activities and Participation describes

a. the ability of the client to execute tasks/activities.
b. the client's highest probable functioning level.
c. whether factors serve as facilitators or barriers.
d. what the client does in the current environment.

75. When documenting a negative event involving a mental-health client, the BEST and legally correct description is

a. "Client rude and obnoxious, spitting at CTRS."
b. "Client screaming 'I hate you ugly freaks' while spitting at CTRSs trying to calm him."
c. "Client disruptive."
d. "Client upset and angry, behaving badly."

76. A card game in which the clients have 5 or 6 cards and must turn over a card if its description ("4 of hearts") is called out is MOST likely used to improve

a. communication.
b. cognitive thinking.
c. memory.
d. concentration.

77. When asked to draw a self-portrait, a client draws a tiny stick figure caught in a giant spider web. The BEST response is for the CTRS to

a. Explain that the client did not follow directions.
b. Ask the reason for drawing the spider web.
c. Discuss the meaning of the spider web with the client.
d. Focus on the stick figure alone.

78. Which of the following horticultural activities is MOST appropriate to promote the use of fine motor skills?

a. Building a dish garden
b. Examining leaves with a magnifying glass
c. Hoeing in the garden
d. Watering potted plants with a hose

79. According to Flow Theory (Csikszentmihalyi), flow occurs when

a. skill level is high and challenge level is low.
b. skill level is high and challenge level is high.
c. skill level is low and challenge level is low.
d. skill level is low and challenge level is high.

80. The primary goal of the recovery model for clients with mental illness is to help the clients to

a. return to the previous level of functioning.
b. avoid relapses and complications.
c. maintain control of their lives and make decisions.
d. maintain treatment protocols.

81. The best response to a client who is progressing well after a stroke but remains extremely fearful and anxious about discharge is to

a. explore the client's concerns with the client.
b. reassure the client that everything will be all right.
c. refer the client to a psychologist.
d. tell the client to call if problems arise after discharge.

82. Which of the following interventions is MOST appropriate for a client with autism and proprioceptive (position and movement) impairment?

a. Walking on a balance beam
b. Jumping on a trampoline
c. Stair walking
d. Wearing a weighted vest

83. Which of the following leisure assessment tools uses pictures of activities to assesses areas of interest in leisure, emotional motivation, and attraction to risk-taking activities?

a. Recreation Behavior Inventory
b. Leisure Activity Blank
c. Leisure Scope
d. Leisure Barriers Inventory

84. The focus of the Medical Model of recreation therapy is on

a. the changes that must occur in the environment.
b. maintaining function at the current level.
c. all people and interactions as therapy.
d. recreation as a clinical treatment.

85. Which of the following forms of therapy is MOST likely to help a client with PTSD express feelings and reduce anxiety?

a. Art therapy
b. Paintball
c. Skeet shooting
d. Soccer

86. A client refuses to make eye contact, is extremely sensitive to sound and touch, communicates poorly with other, and exhibits repetitive behavior. These are characteristics of

a. dementia.
b. autism spectrum disorder.
c. Down syndrome.
d. traumatic brain injury.

87. Once a client has expressed interest in a leisure activity, the CTRS carries out a task/activity analysis, which includes the following steps:

1. assess the client for physical skills required.
2. determine what the client needs to know to participate.
3. separate the activity into component parts.
4. assess what modifications are required.

Which of the following correctly orders these steps from first to last?

a. 1, 2, 3, 4
b. 2, 1, 3, 4
c. 3, 2, 1, 4
d. 1, 3, 4, 2

88. If a client expresses interest in bowling, which of the following physical/mental parameters should the CTRS assess?

a. Patience, endurance, and concentration
b. Vision, hearing, and proprioception
c. Patience, strength, hearing, and endurance
d. Strength, balance, flexibility, and coordination

89. A 70-year-old client is disoriented to time and place, has short-term memory loss, and repeats the same questions over and over but retains motor skills. These indications are MOST likely characteristics of

a. traumatic brain injury.
b. dementia.
c. stroke.
d. depression.

90. The CTRS is planning a wheelchair dance for wheelchair-bound adolescent clients. The PRIMARY concern is

a. the types of dances to include.
b. the use of manual wheelchairs vs motorized.
c. the diagnoses of the clients.
d. the wishes of the clients.

91. A client who was a bicycler has lost vision in both eyes but wants to continue bicycling. The BEST solution is

a. 3-wheeled bicycle.
b. bicycling on an enclosed track.
c. tandem bicycling.
d. stationary bicycling.

92. If the CTRS wants to assess a client's past history of leisure activities and interests in future participation, the MOST appropriate assessment instrument is the

a. Leisure Activity Blank.
b. Recreation Behavior Inventory.
c. Leisure Motivation Scale.
d. Functional Assessment of Characteristics for Therapeutic Recreation.

93. Which of the following is an example of a well-written measurable objective?

a. Following three classes, the client will understand weight loss principles
b. The client will be able to prepare low-calories foods
c. After self-directed study, the client will have knowledge of various weight loss programs and lose weight
d. Following one-on-one instruction about weight loss, the client will be able to list 4 strategies for weight loss

94. A client with cerebral palsy has steadfastly refused to participate in activities the CTRS planned in order to increase the client's strength. The BEST approach is to

a. explain the value of the activity.
b. insist that the client participate.
c. collaborate with the client to find different activities.
d. refer the client to a different CTRS.

95. Which of the following activities is most appropriate for a client with muscular dystrophy and severely limited physical strength?

a. Weight lifting
b. Water therapy
c. Adaptive tennis
d. Tandem bicycling

96. In order to easily follow a client's progress, the BEST documentation format is

a. narrative description.
b. graph.
c. checklist.
d. table.

97. If assessing a client's use of social media and the Internet in the home environment, the INITIAL factor to assess is

a. internet access.
b. interest in social media.
c. computer knowledge.
d. fine motor skills.

98. A discharge plan should include

a. list of coping skills utilized.
b. list of barriers still present at discharge.
c. list of costs associated with activities.
d. list of family and friends.

99. What is the minimum period of internship necessary for the Academic Path to certification from the NCTRC?

a. 6 weeks/240 hours
b. 10 weeks/400 hours
c. 14 weeks/560 hours
d. 20 weeks/800 hours

100. When assessing an older adult with mild cognitive impairment, the CTRS is using the Digit Repetition Test to assess attention. People with normal intelligence (without expressive aphasia) should be able to repeat

a. 3 to 4 numbers.
b. 5 to 7 numbers.
c. 8 to 10 numbers.
d. 11 to 12 numbers.

101. Which of the following professionals is MOST appropriate for a client who is having difficulty swallowing?

a. Nurse practitioner
b. Physical therapist
c. Speech therapist
d. Occupational therapist

102. A client who returned from military service in Afghanistan has begun to have severe frightening flashbacks related to post-traumatic stress syndrome (PTSD). If the CTRS finds the client cowering in the corner of the room in a state of panic, the best approach is to say

a. "Give me your hand and I'll help you up."
b. "I know you are afraid, but you are safe here."
c. "Just deep breathe and relax."
d. "There is nothing to be afraid of."

103. Clients who are diagnosed with severe depression and engaging in recreation therapy as part of treatment should be routinely assessed for

a. functional abilities.
b. risk of falls.
c. suicidal ideation.
d. PTSD.

104. Which of the following patterns of symptoms are characteristic of schizophrenia?

a. Positive symptoms (delusions, hallucinations) or negative symptoms (flat affect, social isolation)
b. Mood swings between depression and mania
c. Impaired social interactions, communication problems, and repetitive behaviors
d. Self-image disturbance, self-mutilating behavior, and fear of abandonment

105. Normalization refers to

a. the client behaving in a normal fashion.
b. the conditions of life being as normal as possible.
c. the client's mental status being stable.
d. the client returning to the home environment.

106. Which of the following assessment tools requires the CTRS to observe a client's behavior in 20 different activities in order to evaluate skills (cognitive, motor, sensory)?

a. Leisure Motivation Scale
b. Recreation Behavior Inventory
c. Leisure Barriers Inventories
d. Leisure Activity Blank

107. If a recreation therapy program focuses on functional interventions to improve both physical and social functioning, which of the following assessments is MOST indicated?

a. Functional
b. Leisure interests
c. Self-esteem
d. Community resources

108. A recreation therapy program includes many different service options. The BEST method of placement to ensure positive outcomes is by

a. client selection.
b. CTRS selection.
c. availability.
d. assessment.

109. Which of the following activities may be used to assess fine motor skills?

a. Lifting the arm from the lap and placing on a table
b. Flexing and extending the elbow
c. Picking up pencils from a table top and placing in a cup
d. Raising the arms over the head while holding weights

110. When developing an appropriate exercise plan for a client anorexia nervosa, the CTRS should avoid discussing which of the following?

a. The fun aspects of exercise
b. Balancing energy input and output
c. The social aspects of exercise
d. The relationship of calories to exercise

111. The primary purpose of licensure is to

a. protect the CTRS professional.
b. provide income to the state.
c. protect the consumer.
d. standardize qualifications.

112. The primary difference between an activity director at a long-term care facility and a CTRS is that the CTRS

a. focuses on leisure activities as therapy.
b. focuses on leisure activities as fun.
c. provides services to all clients.
d. provides general interest activities.

113. Which of the following leisure activities to encourage interaction may be MOST beneficial for a client with autism spectrum disorder who is resistive to interacting with others?

a. Music therapy
b. Video games
c. Basketball
d. Board games

114. Which of the following recreational activities is MOST likely to improve gross motor skills?

a. Making cards
b. Playing Jenga
c. Tossing and catching balls/balloons
d. Sorting beads of various sizes

115. The ecological model of therapeutic recreation addresses

a. needed changes within the environment.
b. the physical and mental needs of the client.
c. the need for community resources.
d. interpersonal skills needed to function effectively.

116. According to the attribution model of recreation therapy, the four factors that determine success or failure are

a. ability, effort, difficulty of task, and luck.
b. intention, attitude, support, and effort.
c. belief, support, confidence, and effort.
d. ability, experience, confidence, and education.

117. Clients are asked who could write out the longest list of answers to simple questions in specified time periods: "How many candy bars can you name?" "How many flowers can you name?" and "How do you feel when you can't do something?" The value of this exercise is that it

a. is a fun competitive exercise.
b. encourages honest expression of feelings.
c. requires little physical activity.
d. requires no training.

118. The four core values of recreation therapy include (1) right to leisure, (2) autonomy, (3) optimal health, and (4)

a. accessibility.
b. inclusion.
c. quality of life.
d. integration.

119. The six steps to ethical decision making (listed below) (per ATRA's Ethics Committee) include:

1. Assess whether an ethical problem is present.
2. Choose an action.
3. Identify alternative actions.
4. Gather facts and information about the situation.
5. Identify consequences associated with alternative actions.
6. Evaluate the selected action.

Which of the following correctly orders these steps from first to last?

a. 1, 4, 2, 3, 5, 6
b. 2, 1, 6, 3, 5, 4
c. 1, 2, 6, 3, 5, 4
d. 4, 1, 3, 5, 2, 6

120 According to the Therapeutic Recreation Outcome Model, if recreation therapy helps a client to communicate better, express emotions, and value participation in recreational activities, which of the behavioral domains have been addressed?

a. Cognitive, social, and physical
b. Cognitive, psychological, and physical
c. Cognitive, psychological, and leisure
d. Social, psychological, and leisure

121. The four criteria for active treatment include (1) prescribed and supervised by a physician, (2) based on assessment and individualized treatment plan, (3) specified duration, intensity and frequency of interventions, and (4)

a. positive outcomes expected.
b. focused on evidence-based practice.
c. discharge planning included.
d. prevention efforts.

122. The APIE process is used to develop a program for each client. APIE stands for

a. action, process, interview, and educate
b. assess, plan, implement, and evaluate.
c. assess, program, interview, and educate.
d. admit, prepare, identify, and evaluation.

123. A type 1, outcome-oriented program is designed to serve

a. adolescent clients.
b. older adult clients.
c. individual clients.
d. large group of clients.

124. Prior to taking a client or clients on an outing, such as to a community event, the CTRS should ensure the availability of

a. a security guard to ensure safety.
b. a client to staff ratio of 2:1.
c. a first aid kit and an emergency plan.
d. spending money for participants.

125. If a client appears intelligent and articulate and follows written directions well but repeatedly asks for oral directions to be repeated, the CTRS should suspect

a. mild cognitive impairment.
b. ADHD.
c. dyslexia.
d. hearing deficit.

126. With reflective listening, if a client is speaking about loss and pauses, the BEST response is to

a. maintain interested silence.
b. ask how the client is feeling.
c. encourage the client to keep talking.
d. ask a question about the previous comments.

127. When assessing a mental health client for affect, if the client's affect is essentially blank and immobile, it would be classified as

a. blunted.
b. flat.
c. inappropriate.
d. bizarre.

128. If a client who is participating in a weight lifting program begins to overtrain, the outcome is likely to be

a. increased performance.
b. decreased performance.
c. no change in performance.
d. burnout.

129. A client agrees to participate in activities but during the activities is sullen and makes frequent complaints. Which type of communication does this represent?

a. Passive-aggressive
b. Assertive
c. Passive
d. Aggressive

130. Under the Individuals with Disabilities Education Act (IDEA) requirements, a functional behavioral assessment (FBA) for children includes assessment of (1) precipitating conditions, (2) specific behavior observed, (3) consequences, and (4)

a. response to consequences.
b. duration of the behavior.
c. function of the behavior.
d. interactions with others.

131. All of the following indicate possible developmental delays for a 6-year-old child EXCEPT

a. inability to catch a ball.
b. poor fine motor skills.
c. speech problems.
d. poor penmanship.

132. If a client does self-assessment with the CAGE tool and answers 2 of the 4 questions with "yes", this indicates

a. no drinking problem.
b. possible drinking problem.
c. drinking problem.
d. severe drinking problem.

133. The primary difference between regular tennis and wheelchair tennis is

a. the ball does not have to bounce within bounds.
b. there is no difference.
c. the ball can bounce three times before being returned.
d. the ball can bounce two times before being returned.

134. The CTRS makes a post-discharge evaluation visit to a client recovering from burn injuries, but the client answers the door and smells of alcohol, slurs words, and swears at the CTRS. Which is the MOST appropriate action?

a. Ask if there is someone else at home with whom the CTRS could speak
b. Call the physician for guidance
c. Reschedule the visit and leave without entering the home
d. Remain supportive, not responding to hostile words, and complete evaluation

135. If a client with chronic alcoholism stops drinking, the first stage of withdrawal usually begins within

a. 4 hours.
b. 8 hours.
c. 12 hours.
d. 24 hours.

136. When providing feedback to a client, all of the following are appropriate EXCEPT

a. be objective and specific.
b. provide suggestions for change/improvement.
c. give negative feedback only in private.
d. compare the client's performance to that of others.

137. When using the CRAFFT screening tool to assess risk-taking behavior in adolescents, the C stands for

a. car.
b. criminal act.
c. creativity.
d. capability.

138. The four stages of recovery from substance abuse/addiction are listed below:

1. Early abstinences.
2. Maintenance.
3. Initiation.
4. Advanced recovery.

Which of the following correctly orders these stages from first to last?

a. 1, 2, 3, 4
b. 3, 1, 2, 4
c. 1, 3, 4, 2
d. 3, 1, 4, 2

139. A client with diabetes mellitus, type 2 (non-insulin dependent) is engaged in walking and jogging. Which of the following focuses of education is MOST important for this client?

a. Foot examination and care
b. Time and duration of exercise
c. Hydration during exercise
d. Diet and nutrition

140. If planning a program for a client and using the person-centered model of care, an essential element to include is

a. community resources.
b. family input.
c. social wellbeing.
d. choice.

141. When developing an individual recreation therapy program for a client with Alzheimer's disease and moderate dementia in a long-term care facility, the MOST important factor to consider is

a. past interests and activities.
b. current cognitive status.
c. input from other staff members.
d. client's attention span.

142. If the CTRS finds that there are no community-based recreational facilities that accommodate clients with disabilities, the CTRS should

a. send letters of complaint about lack of inclusion.
b. provide education and guidance regrading inclusion.
c. begin a petition to force facilities to accommodate inclusion.
d. look for alternatives to community-based recreation.

143. An adolescent hospitalized and under strict isolation may MOST benefit from

a. playing electronic games.
b. watching TV.
c. reading books and magazines.
d. drawing and/or painting.

144. Before children and adolescents with Down syndrome engage in gymnastics or contact sports, it is MOST important to

a. have the cervical spine evaluated by a physician.
b. have the parents sign informed consent.
c. carry out a functional assessment.
d. obtain results of an IQ test.

145. Which of the following is a social barrier to participation in community-based recreational facilities?

a. Client cannot afford private or public transportation
b. Client does not want to share personal information about health
c. Client has no friends to help with transportation
d. Client can't find information and recreational facilities

146. The CTRS at a long-term care facility has obtained a grant to develop an activity room. The FIRST step should be to

a. purchase a variety of supplies and equipment.
b. consult with staff at other facilities with activity rooms.
c. begin with only inexpensive arts and craft supplies.
d. survey clients as to their interests.

147. If clients are participating in a game of basketball in a gym, those with hyperactivity or attention deficit disorders may especially become distressed because of the

a. stress of playing.
b. noise level.
c. energy expended.
d. duration of play.

148. The CTRS has divided the gym into 4 areas for 4 different activities (throwing hoops, badminton, gymnastics, and weight lifting) that are going on at the same time under the CTRS's supervision. This practice

a. makes good use of facilities.
b. reduces staffing costs.
c. increases the risk of injury.
d. violates OSHA guidelines.

149. Which of the following responses is an example of therapeutic communication with a client who states that an activity is too difficult?

a. "Let's talk about how we can make this activity easier for you."
b. "Just hang in there. It will get easier in time."
c. "The other clients seem to have no problem."
d. "What seems to be the problem with the activity?

150. If a client consistently scores 4 in ability to perform tasks on the Functional Independence Measure (FIM), what percentage of the required effort for the task is the client able to achieve?

a. 25%
b. 50%
c. 75%
d. 100%

Answer Key and Explanations

1. B: If the CTRS is encouraging team members to use the STAR approach to client safety, the CTRS explains that the STAR approach includes the following steps:

S	Stop to concentrate on the task at hand.
T	Think about the best way to carry out the task.
A	Act to accomplish the necessary task.
R	Review the success of or problems with the task completion.

2. A: If a client with a history of aggression begins swearing and pacing back and forth, yelling, "You can't make me stay here!" the best initial response is to speak calmly and quietly to the client. The CTRS should remain in control and avoid reactions that suggest fear or anger. The CTRS should stand if sitting but avoid moving aggressively toward the client but should move toward the door if the situation appears to be escalating and it is safe to do so.

3. D: Confirmability. In evaluating research as part of the development of evidence-based practice guidelines, the four evaluative/trustworthiness criteria are:

- Credibility: Documentation supports accuracy and validity.
- Dependability: Evidence shows how conclusions are reached and whether others should expect to each the same conclusions.
- Transferability: The extent to which the results can apply to others in similar situations.
- Confirmability: The data are clear and show how conclusions are reached.

4. A: If a client with multiple sclerosis tells the CTRS that she is upset that she can no longer continue her employment because her job is too physically demanding and is concerned about how she will support herself, the response that focuses on problem solving as a response to stress is "What options have you considered for less physically demanding work?" This response doesn't suggest a solution, such as public assistance, but indirectly suggests that the client can take control to solve the problem of work.

5. B: The Joint Commission requires two identifiers to ensure that the correct individual is receiving care and that the care is intended for that individual. Identifiers must be specific to the client. The first identifier is usually the client's name, often found on the wristband, and the second can be the birthdate, client ID number, or telephone number. Birthplace is usually too non-specific as is place of employment. If an armband is used as an identifier, it must be on the client's body and cannot be simply placed at bedside or taped to a bedside stand.

6. A: 4- to 5-year-olds may participate in dancing, skating and other supervised activities but lack coordination and judgment about safety. 6- to 12-year-olds are still growing and muscles are short, so they do best with non-competitive sports, such as bicycling and swimming, until about age 10. Team sports should be supervised to ensure children are not straining muscles. Weight lifting may be done at 11. Gymnastics may begin with children monitored for eating disorders. 12- to 18-year-olds can participate in any sports activity unless limited by illness or disability.

7. A: A cost-benefit analysis uses average cost of a problem and the cost of intervention to demonstrate savings and to determine if an intervention is a sound investment. For example, if the lack of CTRS at an organization results in $80,000 loss of income each year and hiring a CTRS costs $40,000 in salary and $16,000 in benefits for a total of $56,000, the cost benefit is calculated by subtracting the intervention costs from the annual loss: $80,000 – 56,000 = $24,000. If the calculation results in a negative number, then there is no benefit.

8. C: 4, 1, 3, 2, 5. The stages of substance abuse include:

- Experimentation: Use is occasional in social settings or in response to stressful situations.
- Regular use: A regular pattern of use emerges.
- Problem use: The person experiences problems because of substance abuse.
- Dependence: The person continues chronic use despite problems and risks and exhibits increasing tolerance and withdrawal.
- Addiction: The person feels a physical and psychological need for the substance, despite problems it is causing, experiences cravings, and exhibits alcohol/drug seeking behaviors.

9. D: Characteristics that indicate a dog is likely well-suited to be a therapy dog include:

- Remains confident in different environment.
- Likes to meet people (but is not overly enthusiastic or excited).
- Remains well-controlled and calm.
- Is mature (past the puppy stage) and psychological sound.
- Comfortable with people who act differently.

While trained dogs are preferred, they are not required. Many dogs, depending on training and temperament, may serve as therapy dogs. Some characteristics are warning signs: fearfulness, excitability, aggressiveness, poor heath, guarding of toys and food, and licking of people.

10. A: If when utilizing the Plan-Do-Study-Act (PDSA) method of continuous quality improvement, study of the outcomes of a trial indicates that the solution that was instituted was not effective, the next step is to return to the Plan step in order to select a different solution. Method:

- Plan: Define the problem, brainstorm, and collect data.
- Do: Generate solutions, choose one, and implement a trial.
- Study: Evaluate outcomes.
- Act: Identify changes needed for full implementation and continue to monitor.

11. B: While these are all important steps, the first step should be to consider the source and to eliminate articles in the popular press and to focus on juried articles in medical journals to avoid wasting time on articles that lack validity and reliability. Next, the author's credentials should be reviewed to determine if the author is an expert in the field or has the proper credentials to write with authority about the topic.

12. A: The three primary elements of motivational interviewing, which focuses on the role motivation has in bringing about change in an individual, are:

- Collaboration: Working with the client rather than confronting the client in order to resolve issues.
- Evocation: Drawing out ideas from the client about problems and solutions rather than imposing ideas of the interviewer.
- Autonomy: Recognizing that the client is the one who is responsible for making changes and respecting the client's choices.

13. D: When entering the examining room of a client who is deaf and facing away from the door, the CTRS should clap or tap the foot. Clients who are deaf are often more sensitive to vibrations, so this will likely alert them that someone is present. If there is no response, the CTRS should try to approach from the direction the client is facing in order to avoid startling the client by touching the client from behind.

14. C: If an adverse incident occurs, a written report should be completed immediately or as soon as possible. The adverse incident report should include the names of those involved or witnessing the incident, identifying information, time, date, and location, and a narrative description of what happened, actions taken at the time or subsequent to the incident. Each organization should have established protocols for documenting adverse incidents, and the CTRS should follow the protocol.

15. A: The greatest barrier to communication is a condition in which the client is extremely anxious and crying. Clients who are distressed have very poor retention because of the inability to concentrate. This poses a bigger problem than mild cognitive impairment (MCI), which often involves poor short-term memory. Clients with MCI may need to have information written down to help with their retention or may need reminders. Hearing and vision impairments do not necessarily result in barriers to communication.

16. B: The best method of ensuring that a client follows the plan of care is to include the client in the planning. If possible, the client should actively participate in developing a problem list and should have input into the most appropriate interventions and expected outcomes. Clients are less likely to cooperate if a plan of care is imposed on them, especially if they don't understand the benefits of the plan.

17. B: If the CTRS has called a client who is being treated for chronic depression because the client has missed one appointment and two sessions of the support group, the statement by the client that is of most concern is: "I've been giving all my things away, and I feel so much better." Clients suffering from depression who decide to commit suicide often begin to give away their things and claim that they feel better, and may even appear calmer and more relaxed, but these are warning signs.

18. A: If a stroke client has been discharged home but is having difficulty preparing foods because of residual right-sided weakness, the most appropriate referral is to an occupational therapist. Occupational therapists can help the client with exercises to increase strength in the right hand and can also show the client how to compensate for the right-sided weakness and how to use assistive devices in order to cook safely.

19. D: A nonverbal clue that a client may be anxious is if the client rubs the hands together constantly as this is a self-comforting measure. Nonverbal behavior can include the tone of voice and cadence of speech, body positioning or behaviors (arms crossed, sitting forward, leaning backward), facial expressions (frowning, grimacing, relaxed), eye cast, amount of eye contact, obvious autonomic physiological responses (diaphoresis and blushing), personal appearance (grooming, hygiene), and physical characteristics (extreme over- or under-weight).

20. C: When the CTRS is assisting a nonambulatory client to transfer from a wheelchair into an automobile, the best assistive device is likely a sliding board. Newer sliding boards have a round disc on which the client is seated, and this disc then slides along the board so that the friction during transfer is not on the client's tissue. Slip sheets are used to reposition clients. The lateral transfer device aids in lateral transfers, such as from the bed to a gurney. Transfer/Pivot discs are circular discs on which a client stands and is then pivoted to sit.

21. C: If a CTRS dislikes working with older adults and frequently avoids older clients while showing favoritism to young adults of a similar age to the CTRS, this is an example of a boundary violation. While CTRS are allowed personal preferences, they should not act on these preferences and allow these preferences to influence the care they provide. Showing favoritism is a failure to maintain a therapeutic relationship and does not serve the needs of the clients.

22. A: If when interviewing a client whose culture is different from the CTRS, the CTRS asks what the client believes is the cause of the client's symptoms and what treatment the client expects, this is an example of cultural competence. The CTRS recognizes that clients from different cultures may have very different ideas about the causes of disease and the appropriate response than is typical in Western society. It's important to understand the client's frame of reference.

23. D: The primary purpose of conducting a problem-based assessment on a client is to create a problem list based on a thorough exam and history. Once a list of problems is identified, then the problems are prioritized so that the most critical issues are dealt with first. One problem may involve a number of different physical and psychosocial elements. For example, poor nutrition may relate to the inability to physically prepare food, depression, inadequate resources to purchase nutritious food, and lack of transportation.

24. D: Performing. Tuckman's stages include:

- Forming: The leader lists the goals and rules and encourages communication.
- Storming: A divergence of opinions regarding management, power, and authority may lead to increased stress and resistance with absence of members, shared silence, and subgroup formation.
- Norming: Members express positive feelings toward each other and feel deeply attached to the group.
- Performing: The leader's input and direction decreases and mainly consists of keeping the group on course.
- Mourning: This is most deeply felt in closed groups when discontinuation of the group nears and in open groups when the leader or other members leave.

25. A: The four components of the Therapeutic Service Delivery Model (Van Andel) include (1) Diagnosis/Needs assessment, (2) Treatment/Rehabilitation, (3) Education, and (4) Prevention/Health Promotion. Service is provided in a continuum from acute care to community-based programs. The interactions between the client and the CTRS begin with the client giving informed consent to treatment and continue along the path to the client being able to make rational choices about actions and to act independently.

26. D: The primary goals of client advocacy are to promote client independence by encouraging self-care and recognizing the right to self-determination and to promote improvement in the healthcare system by supporting professional organizations, communicating with administrators and legislators, lobbying, assessing needs of the community, planning programs, and implementing change. The CTRS must educate the client about services and help the client to actively participate and make decisions about care. The CTRS may serve as an advocate by introducing interventions to help to decrease barriers to care.

27. B: Clients who undergo amputations often experience Kübler-Ross's five stages of grief associated with death and other losses as they try to cope with physical disability and changes in their body image. During the stage of denial, clients may believe unrealistically that they need no assistance and can return to their routine lives with no problem. Other stages include anger, bargaining, depression, and acceptance. Clients may not go through all stages or may go through the stages in no particular order.

28. C: While all of these are important, preventing complications after a spinal cord injury is critical because development of complications may severely limit independence and impair psychological wellbeing and may be life-threatening. Common complications include pressure sores, urinary tract infections, deep vein thrombosis, pulmonary emboli, pneumonia, and autonomic dysreflexia. Pressure sores can lead to severe systemic infection. Heterotropic ossification (development of bone in soft tissue), especially of the hips, can be overlooked until it is advanced but can result in impaired range of motion and mobility.

29. C: A point of service plan is a structure that combines aspects of an HMO with a PPO. Clients are able to receive care from healthcare providers within the network or may seek treatment outside the network in some circumstances. This type of plan offers more flexibility to the client, but usually there are additional costs when a client chooses to seek treatment outside of the network. Co-payments may increase and the percentage of costs covered by the plan may decrease.

30. A: A bipolar client who is very nervous about transitioning into the community from a sheltered environment may benefit from a support group comprised of people dealing with similar issues. Support groups may have a mental health professional as a leader. Support groups are usually open groups that allow clients to choose whether or not to attend, but the groups provide a safe and supportive atmosphere where people can discuss shared concerns and methods of coping.

31. C: Because of perceived excess costs associated with recreational, occupational, physical, and speech therapy, careful documentation must include realistic and measurable goals as well as a physician's order for therapy and evidence that therapy was provided by or supervised by a licensed therapist who conducted a thorough evaluation and developed a plan of care that included frequency and duration of treatment. Documentation must also indicate that the therapy was medically necessary. The same documentation requirements apply to skilled nursing facilities.

32. A: Problem-solving involves actively searching for a way to reduce stress and cope. Avoidance means to avoid stressors or reduce their impact if possible. Physical activity can often increase feelings of wellbeing and allow people to cope more effectively. Spirituality can involve attending religious services or engaging in religious or spiritual endeavors to provide emotional support and a positive outlook. Those with ineffective coping skills may express anxiety, anger, and agitation (which may interfere with decision making) and may develop depression and physical ailments, such as anorexia, weight loss, nausea, urinary and bowel problems, and sleep disturbance.

33. B: The CTRS should immediately place the client on a second shelter waiting list to increase the chance for placement even though the client may prefer a different shelter. Discharging a client into the streets poses an ethical dilemma, and if no placement can be found, then Social Services may be able to provide some alternatives. The decision about calling daily depends on the individual shelter and the relationship the CTRS has with the shelter administration. Transferring to a level of care that is higher than needed is not a viable option even with Medicaid, and the client is indigent and uninsured.

34. B: Assistive devices include shower chairs, handrails, adaptive kitchen equipment, ostomy and wound care supplies. Basic mobility aids include crutches, canes, and walkers. Mobility aids include wheelchairs, scooter, seat-lift cushions, and electric beds. High-technology equipment includes apnea/sleep monitors, ventilators, parenteral/enteral nutrition, infusion pumps, and specialized electronic/computerized equipment for quadriplegia/paraplegia. Durable medical equipment must be approved, and Medicare regulations require the equipment be purchased from a Medicare-participating supplier.

35. C: The CTRS should not interrupt a child at play with a direct question, which interferes with the child's process of working out feelings of anxiety and may cause increased stress. A better approach is to use a reflective statement, such as "I see that the little boy in your picture is crying" or "I wonder why the little boy is crying," and leave it to the child to respond or not. Focusing on the picture rather than the child may be less threatening and help the child to explain why the child in the picture is crying.

36. A: "The law doesn't allow me to give out any information about clients in order to protect their privacy and safety" is accurate and appropriate. The Health Insurance Portability and Accountability Act (HIPAA) addresses the privacy of health information. It is essential to never release any information or documentation about a client's condition or treatment without consent. Personal information about the client is considered protected health information (PHI), and it includes any identifying or personal information about the client, such as health history, condition, or treatments in any form, and any documentation. Failure to comply with HIPAA regulations can make one liable for legal action.

37. D: Many people are more sensitive to sensory overload in the afternoon when cortisol levels are highest. Sensory overload most often affects those with cognitive impairment or those in stressful situations. Excess noise and activity can cause distress, agitation, increase confusion, and delirium. Sensory deprivation occurs when there is too little environmental stimulation because of reduction in sensory input because of hearing or vision deficits, inability to recognize sensory input because of cognitive impairment, or boring environment. Sensory deprivation can contribute to confusion, disorientation, and depression.

38. B: Physiological needs must be met first. Maslow stated that human behavior is motivated by needs and that there is a hierarchy of needs that begin with basic needs and progress to personal needs. The hierarchy includes:

- Physiological needs (the base).
- Safety and security.
- Belonging.
- Self-esteem.
- Self-actualization (the apex).

People may not progress in one direction from one need to another but movement may be in multiple directions in a lifelong process of working toward self-actualization, which requires creativity and some degree of freedom. Failure to develop toward self-actualization may result in depression and feelings of failure.

39. C: Assessing family dynamics is not a primary goal of using play therapeutically. Goals include establishing contact with the child, observing the child's behavior and interactions and collecting data, and interpreting the child's behavior based on those observations. For this type of assessment, the CTRS should choose simple play items that can be used by the child in a number of different ways, such as blocks, paper and crayons, dolls, cars, and clay. Familiar toys may provide a sense of comfort to the child.

40. C: Children should engage in healthcare play in which they provide treatment with dolls or stuffed animals and never other children or adults. Children, especially those who have been hurt by procedures, are often quite aggressive during play and could potentially hurt someone standing in as "patient" during the play, such as by jabbing the person hard with a needle-less syringe. Additionally, the child may be inhibited by play with another person while a doll, for example, provides a passive participant.

41. A: Assessment of a client's level of interest in activities should include the type of activity, past interest (10 years), recent interest (1 year), current participation, and future interest in participation in order to gain a full picture. Reviewing a checklist of activities with the client is better than simply asking about activities because recall may be better than production. Activities of interest in the past provide valuable information because sometimes clients stop activities because of disabilities rather than lack of interest. Current participation and future interests are especially important in planning interventions.

42. A: Because of autonomic nervous system dysfunction, thermoregulation (including sweating) is impaired, so hyperthermia (overheating) is of great concern in high temperature. Body temperature fluctuates according to ambient temperature, even in the shade. Clients with injuries higher than T6 are especially at risk. The client may readily develop signs of heat stress or even heat stroke, so clients should be advised to keep a cool damp cloth around the neck, mist the face and neck with cool water, remain hydrated, and wear light, non-constricting clothing.

43. D: Role modeling is a central concept to Bandura's (1977, 2001) Social Learning Theory with mentoring an example. The learner may perceive and interpret input in different ways. This theory stresses that the attitudes and behavior of the educators and staff influence the outcomes of the learners. Bandura stated that social learning is primarily an internal process with four steps: attentional phase (observing a role model), retention phase (processing information), reproduction phase (memory utilized to guide performance of role model's actions) and motivational phase (vicarious reinforcement and punishment).

44. A: The first step in conducting a program evaluation is to determine the purpose of the evaluation and then to establish a time frame (formative or summative) and decide when to evaluate and who will do the evaluations. The design of the evaluation is an important consideration and may involve selecting or creating an evaluation instrument. Data must be collected and interpreted with the results reported and used to make decisions. Costs of evaluation must be considered as well.

45. B: If using the DARP focused charting format, DARP stands for:

- Data: Includes the focus of the problem with objective observations as well as subjective complaints: "Client complains of anxiety. Face flushed, rubbing hands together frequently, and pacing back and forth."
- Action: Interventions necessary to resolve the problem: "Practiced deep breathing and relaxation exercises with visualization for 20 minutes and listened to classical music."
- Response: Reactions to action taken: "Client sitting quietly, color normal."
- Plan: Preventive measures: "Assist client with coping strategies."

46. C: A client who needs low impact physical exercise may benefit from water aerobics because the water's buoyancy diminishes impact and protects the joints. Both running in place and playing tennis are high impact activities because both feet may be off the ground at one time. With low impact, only one foot is usually off the ground at a time, so this may include walking and hill climbing. No impact activities may include bicycling and swimming.

47. D: The Experiential Learning Theory (Kolb) suggests that divergent learners like to work with people:

- Divergent: Prefers concrete experience and reflective observations and is imaginative with good ideas and is emotional. Likes working with people.
- Accommodative: Prefers a combination of concrete experience and active experimentation, solves problems through trial and error, and tends to complete tasks.
- Assimilative: Prefers abstract concepts and reflective observation and is more interested in abstract ideas than people and applying ideas.
- Convergent: Prefers abstract concepts and active experimentation and prefers dealing with things to people.

48. B: The Americans with Disabilities Act requires that recreation parks and facilities provide access to the disabled, including removal of architectural barriers. The ADA regulations apply to a variety of facilities: amusement rides, exercise equipment, boating facilities, piers for fishing, golf, mini-golf, children's playgrounds and play areas, shooting galleries/facilities, spa/fitness centers, and swimming pools. Additionally, the ADA includes guidelines for outdoor recreational areas.

49. A: The Instrumental Activities of Daily Living instrument does not assess bathing or the ability to carry out personal hygiene. The AIDL includes assessment of:

- Telephone use.
- Shopping for food, clothes, or needed items.
- Food preparation, diet plan.
- Housekeeping, including all household duties.
- Laundry.
- Transportation availability.
- Medications, ability to manage prescriptions and taking medications.
- Financial responsibility, budget, pay bills.

50. D: In order to receive accreditation from the Commission on Accreditation of Rehabilitation Facilities (CARF), the most important responsibility is to conform to internationally accepted standards. provides voluntary accreditation to health and human service organizations, such as aging services, behavioral health, medical rehabilitation, opioid treatment programs, and child and youth services. Accreditation requires consultation with CARF resource specialist for assistance with preparation, self-evaluation, application, payment of a fee, and a survey by CARF surveyors. Accreditation may be provisional or for one to three years.

51. C: The goal of the Leisure Ability Model of treatment is for the client to become increasingly independent in treatment/activities. While the client may be dependent on the CTRS at the beginning of therapy, the client should assume more and more responsibility and make decisions about leisure activities that promote independence and a feeling of wellbeing. The CTRS serves as a therapist, counselor, and resource person helping the client to improve functional behavior and make choices to overcome barriers and to fully participate in activities. The model progresses from treatment to leisure education and recreation participation.

52. C: Community inclusion services is a specialization recognized by the NCTRC. Additional specialization areas include adaptive sports and recreation, behavioral health, developmental disabilities, geriatrics, pediatrics, and physical medicine/rehabilitation. A designation of specialization on the credential indicates that the CTRS has completed continuing education and/or has experience in a specialized area. The specialization designation is current for 5 years.

53. B: Under the Individual with Disabilities Education Act, therapeutic recreation is generally indicated as a related service. Related services are those that are supportive and allow the child to participate in an individualized education program. Other related services include transportation services, psychological counseling, physical therapy, audiology, occupation therapy, mobility services, speech therapy, and social work services.

54. A: Characteristics consistent with addictive personalities include:

- Impulsive: Do not think of consequences.
- Thrill-seeking: Enjoy the dopamine-powered rush.
- Lying: Often lie to cover up addictions.
- Stressed: Stress of needing a fix/drink and inability to obtain it.
- History of personal or family addiction: Increases risk that the client will be attracted to or resume addictions.

55. D: According to the Self-Determination Theory (Ryan and Deci), intrinsic motivation is diminished by external rewards (because they take the focus away from the self) and by threats or coercion. Intrinsic motivation is stimulated by nurturing the client's wishes/desires, considering the client's needs when structuring activities/lessons, encouraging active participation and autonomy, providing positive feedback, acknowledging client's frustrations/negative responses, and providing choices.

56. C: If a client who wants to play table tennis again after an injury has poor manual strength and limited dexterity, the best solution is likely utilizing an adaptive glove that facilitates gripping of the table tennis paddle. While video simulation may be available or other activities easier, therapy should be guided by what the client wants to do because this supports the client's motivation and sense of achievement.

57. C: If the CTRS is applying for recertification under option 1, the CTRS must have completed 480 hours of work in the field and 50 hours of continuing education related to topics listed in the job analysis carried out by NCTRC. The CTRS may also choose to recertify by passing the national certification exam, which is administered twice yearly and can be completed online. The cost of recertification is $25 plus $80 maintenance fee. There is also a continuing education approval process review fee of $35.

58. B: An essential element of mentoring is providing feedback: Being honest in evaluation and assisting others to improve, providing feedback about how their practices affect client outcomes. Other elements include:

- Nurturing: Being supportive and interested in furthering the skills and education of the staff.
- Providing clinical expertise: Guiding by demonstrating a personal commitment to excellence.
- Motivating others: Encouraging others and supporting them throughout their careers.
- Providing an example: Teaching others by being a good example.
- Listening: Being non-judgmental in discussions with others and listening to determine different perspectives and needs.
- Role modeling: Providing assistance to others in gaining certification and understanding the role of CTRS.

59. A: According to Principle 9 (Competence) of the ATRA Code of Ethics, the CTRS is responsible for continually seeking to expand knowledge in recreation therapy. The Code of Ethics contains 10 principles: (1) Beneficence, (2) Non-maleficence, (3) Autonomy, (4) Justice, (5) Fidelity, (6) Veracity, (7) Informed Consent, (8) Confidentiality and Privacy, (9) Competence, and (10) Compliance with Laws and Regulations.

60. A: If the CTRS is interested in working with an intern in the field of recreation therapy, the best marketing method is likely to send a latter/email to schools with recreation therapy programs. Many students are unsure where to seek internships, and in some areas, internships can be difficult to find, so those who contact schools and let them know of their interest can often pull from a large pool of students.

61. D: Utilization review assesses the necessity of care in relation to admission, treatment, and discharge as well as adherence to critical pathways. It is used to evaluate whether decision-making, care, and length of treatment are appropriate. Utilization review may be conducted by third-party payors, such as insurance companies. Issues considered during UR include the severity of condition, based on symptoms, history, and testing, and the intensity of service, based on interventions and treatments.

62. B: 2, 1, 4, 3. Risk management is a formal method of decreasing liability, financial loss, and risk or harm to clients, staff, or others by doing an assessment of risk and introducing risk management strategies. Steps include:

- Risk identification: assessment of processes to identify and prioritize those that require further study to determine risk exposure.
- Risk analysis: careful documenting of process, utilizing flow charts, with each step in the process assessed for potential risks.
- Risk prevention: carrying out corrective or preventive processes.
- Assessment/evaluation: ongoing to determine if efforts are effective or require modification.

63. C: The four elements of intervention that are of primary importance in the therapeutic recreation accountability model (TRAM) include assessment implementation, treatment plans, progress notes (documentation), and discharge/referral summaries. TRAM aims to focus on both accountability and documentation and stresses the importance of the program design and the assessment of the client in order to achieve optimal client outcomes. The assessment instrument should adequately match the contents of the program for more accurate placement and development of a treatment plan.

64. A: If someone has made a verbal complaint about a grievance to the program director but believes the response was inadequate, the next step should be to file a formal written complaint to the director or the board (depending on the formal grievance policy that is in place) within a prescribed period of time, usually 30 days. Generally, the director and/or board has 30 days to respond, during which time they conduct an investigation and reach a conclusion.

65. D: Gross negligence. Type of negligence include:

- Negligent conduct: Failure to provide reasonable care or to protect/assist another, based on standards and expertise.
- Gross negligence: Willful provision of inadequate care with disregard for the safety and security of another.

- Contributory negligence: Injured party contributes to his/her own harm.
- Comparative negligence: Attributes percentage amount of negligence to each individual involved.

66. B: The primary advantage of just-in-time ordering of inventory is cost saving. Ordering is done only when the supply of an item is almost depleted, so less money is tied up in inventory on hand. Additionally, there is less chance that supplies will become outdated so there is less loss. Ordering may also be done automatically when a stock item reaches a certain level, especially when inventory is computerized, saving both time and labor.

67. A: Types of budgets:

- Operating: Finances daily operations and includes general expenses, such as salaries, education, insurance, maintenance, depreciation, debts, and profit.
- Capital: Earmarks capital projects (such as remodeling, maintenance repairing, purchasing or upgrading of equipment or facilities).
- Cash balance: Projects cash balances for a specific future time period, including all operating and capital budget items.
- Master: Combines operating, capital, and cash balance budgets as well as any specialized or area-specific budgets.

68. B: If a CTRS is to undergo peer review, the CTRS should expect that the review will be carried out by a CTRS with similar work experience. The peer may or may not be from the same unit/department or organization. The ranking system usually for review includes:

- Care is based on standards and typical of that provided by like practitioners.
- Variance may occur in care, but outcomes are satisfactory.
- Care is not consistent with that provided by like practitioners.
- Variance resulted in negative outcomes.

69. A: When supervising another staff member, the CTRS should focus on what the person is doing correctly because doing so helps the other person to build confidence in his/her own abilities. This does not mean that what the person is doing incorrectly should be ignored (especially if it may compromise client care) but should be dealt with as an area that needs improvement or as an educational need.

70. D: The Health Protection/Health Promotion Model (Pender) suggests that a client's health behavior is influenced by 8 beliefs:

- Perceived benefits: Positive outcomes.
- Perceived barriers: Roadblocks and personal cost.
- Perceived ability to overcome barriers: Degree of self-confidence.
- Activity-associated affect (feelings associated with actions).
- Interpersonal influences: Family, friends, caregivers, role models, social norms, social support.
- Situational influences: How actions fit into lifestyle, environment.
- Commitment to taking action: Motivation and intentions.
- Competing demands/preferences: Alternate forms of behavior.

71. C: 4, 1, 3, 5, 2. Steps to clinical problem solving:

- Define the issue: Talking with those involved to determine if the problem related to a failure of communication or other issues.
- Collect data: Includes interviewing additional staff or reviewing documentation, gaining a variety of perspectives.
- Identify important concepts: Determining if there are issues related to values or beliefs.
- Consider reasons for actions: Distinguishing between motivation and intention on the part of all parties to determine the reason for the problem.
- Make decision: Reaching a decision to prevent a recurrence of a problem based on advocacy and moral agency.

72. A: The solution that is the most appropriate for a visually-impaired client who wants to participate in team sports, such as baseball, is a beeper ball. The foam ball reduces the risk of injury from impact and beeps to provide auditory stimulation so that the visually impaired person can use the sound to locate the ball and follow its movements. The beeper ball can be used with mixed groups with some with and others without visual impairments.

73. B: The primary purpose of palliative care is to relieve pain and discomfort and to improve the quality of life. Palliative care may be offered at any time during the progression of a disease, not necessarily only at the end-of-life. Palliative care may also be provided while a client is actively seeking curative treatment. Palliative care serves may include educating the client about available services and assisting with exercise programs to increase strength and improve mobility.

74. D: The International Classification of Functioning (WHO) is a system for classifying a client's functional abilities. Qualifiers are the means of assessment. The performance qualifier for Activities and Participation describes what the client does in the current environment. Elements of classification include:

- Body functions: Level of impairment.
- Activities and Participation: Performance qualifier as above; capacity qualifier describes the ability to execute tasks/activities.
- Environmental: Assessment of environmental factors.
- Body structures: Level/Degree of impairment.

75. B: Documentation should be as specific and detailed as possible: "Client screaming, 'I hate you ugly freaks' while spitting at CTRSs trying to calm him." The CTRS should avoid judgmental statements, such as "rude and obnoxious," which may be considered defamation of character, specifically libel as it is in written form as opposed to slander, which is oral defamation. "Client disruptive" is too vague and "Client upset and angry, behaving badly" is again making judgments but lacking adequate description.

76. D: A card game in which the clients have 5 or 6 cards and must turn over a card if its description ("4 of hearts") is called out is most likely used to improve concentration. This game can be played with a group of clients. They must pay attention to their cards, listen to the descriptions, determine if the descriptions match their cards, and respond to a match by carrying out an action (turning over the card). The first client to turn over all cards is the game winner.

77. C: If, when asked to draw a self-portrait, a client draws a tiny stick figure caught in a giant spider web, the best response is for the CTRS to discuss the meaning of the spider web with the client, making observations and avoiding direct questioning when possible: "The spider web must have meaning for you. Do you feel like talking about that?" or "I notice that your body size is quite small and the spider web is huge."

78. A: The horticultural activity that is most appropriate to promote the use of fine motor skills is building a dish garden. The client must gather a number of different supplies and small plants, fill the dish with potting soil, and individually place the small plants in the soil. Some dish gardens may also contain small stones or other decorations that must be carefully placed. All of these activities require fine motor skills and help to improve dexterity.

79. B: According to Flow Theory (Csikszentmihalyi), mental states can help or hinder learning, and flow occurs when skill level is high and challenge level is high. A mismatch between skill level and challenge may result in boredom or apathy (if skill level is too high for challenge) or stress and anxiety (if skill level is too low for challenge), so the appropriate balance must be reached in order to attain flow, which is the mental state most conducive to learning.

80. C: The primary goal of the recovery model for clients with mental illness is to help the clients to maintain control of their lives and make decisions. Because some clients may never be able to return to previous levels of functioning, having this as a goal of therapy may result in frustration and increased stress. The recovery model stresses the importance of self-determination and the skills and resilience the clients can draw on in recovery.

81. A: The best response to a client who is progressing well after a stroke (or any illness/injury) but remains extremely fearful and anxious about discharge is to explore the client's concerns with the client, allowing the client to express his or her feelings. The person may have valid reasons for concerns, such as living alone or lack of transportation, and may not fully understand the services that are available in the community or may feel overwhelmed by changes in physical condition and abilities.

82. B: A client with autism and proprioceptive (position and movement) impairment may benefit from activities that involves both movement and changes in position, such as swinging or jumping on a trampoline. Walking on a balance beam, stair walking, and wearing a weighted vest are all interventions that may be utilized to help maintain balance. Weighted vests or snug clothing are also comforting to those with autism who are sensitive to touch and textures.

83. C: Leisure Scope is an assessment tool that uses pictures of activities to assesses areas of interest in leisure, emotional motivation, and attraction to risk-taking activities. Leisure Scope is intended for adults, but a version for adolescents is also available. The instrument takes about 20 minutes to administer (the client chooses between two pictures at a time) and is intended for clients with the cognitive ability of at least a 6-year-old and a Ranchos Los Amigos core of ≥6.

84. D: The focus of the Medical Model of recreation therapy is on recreation as a clinical treatment to address specific health problems. Treatment is prescribed by a physician and begins under direction of the CTRS with the client taking more control of activities as time passes and the client gains confidence. The goal is for the client to go from a state of poor health to good health and to participate in self-directed leisure activities.

85. A: Art therapy is most likely to help a client with PTSD express feelings and reduce anxiety because it is generally carried out in a calm environment and the art work produced by the client can lead to discussions about its meaning. High energy activities, such as paintball and soccer, are sometimes used to transition soldiers from being in a war zone to being at home and may help to prevent PTSD.

86. B: If a client refuses to make eye contact, is extremely sensitive to sound and touch, communicates poorly with others, and exhibits repetitive behavior, these are characteristics of autism spectrum disorder. ASD is characterized by impairment of social interactions (inability to establish friendships or express emotions), impairment of communication (inability to understand nonverbal communication, language delay), and restrictive repetitive or stereotyped behavior (head banging, preoccupation with specific items/topics, and inflexibility).

87. C: 3, 2, 1, 4. Once a client has expressed interest in a leisure activity, the CTRS (1) carries out a task/activity analysis by first separating the activity into component parts and then arranging these components sequentially in order to (2) determine what the client needs to know first in order to participate and then next and so on. After the component parts are identified, the client should be (3) assessed for the physical skills necessary for participation and (4) any limitations that may require modifications or adaptations.

88. D: If a client expresses interest in bowling the physical/mental parameters that the CTRS should assess include:

- Strength: Assessment of hand grip and ability to hold and swing a ball that can weigh up to 16 pounds, depending on the client's age and size.
- Balance: Assessment of ability to walk and slide.
- Flexibility: Assessment of shoulder and arm range of motion to determine ability to deliver the bowling ball.
- Endurance: Assessment of energy levels and ability to maintain participation over the course of a game.

89. B: If a 70-year-old client is disoriented to time and place, has short-term memory loss, and repeats the same questions over and over but retains motor skills, these indications are most likely characteristics of dementia and Alzheimer's disease. The stages of Alzheimer's include: (1) no outward signs, (2) very mild cognitive decline, forgetfulness, (3) short-term memory loss, problem with planning and organizing, (4) moderate cognitive impairment, withdrawal from social activities, (5) moderately severe cognitive impairment with obvious confusion and disorientation, (6) profound confusion, and (7) very severe cognitive impairment, bedbound, incontinent, aphasic.

90. D: If the CTRS is planning a wheelchair dance for wheelchair-bound adolescent clients, the primary concern is the wishes of the clients, who should be actively involved in the planning process and should make the decisions about the types of dances to include. Both manual and motorized wheelchairs can participate in wheelchair dancing, and clients may benefit regardless of diagnosis. Wheelchair dancing may improve strength (especially with manual wheelchairs), improve memory and sequencing abilities (mastering dance moves), and increase socialization.

91. C: If a client who was a bicycler has lost vision in both eyes but wants to continue bicycling, the best solution is tandem bicycling in which a person with vision is the pilot and sits in the front and the vision-impaired person sits in the back. Tandem bicycling allows the vision-impaired person to safely continue with a sport activity outdoors and to still gain the same benefits, such as pleasure, strength, and endurance.

92. A: If the CTRS wants to assess a client's past history of leisure activities and interests in future participation, the most appropriate assessment instrument is the Leisure Activity Blank. LAB helps to assess the types and degrees of activity the client participated in prior to disability and can serve as a guide for selecting leisure activities that the client may enjoy. Because the instrument focuses on both the past and the future, the CTRS can assess how the client's expectations have changed.

93. D: An example of a well-written measurable objective is: "Following one-on-one instruction about weight loss, the client will be able to list 4 strategies for weight loss." The four-part method is often used to write effective specific objectives, which are not only prescriptive but also measurable:

- Condition/Testing circumstance: "Following one-on-one instruction about weight loss"
- Learner: "the client"
- Performance: "will be able to list"
- Criterion: "4 strategies for weight loss."

94. C: If a client with cerebral palsy has steadfastly refused to participate in activities the CTRS planned in order to increase the client's strength, the best approach is to collaborate with the client to find different activities. A plan of treatment should be continually reassessed and modified as needed based on client's participation and response. Clients often feel a lack of control and may express their frustration by refusing to cooperate.

95. B: The activity that is most appropriate for a client with muscular dystrophy and severely limited physical strength is water therapy. Because of the buoyancy of the water, the client may be able to move more than when out of the water, and the water (if warm) may help to relax the client's muscles. Additionally, water activities are low or no impact, so they do not stress the muscles and joints.

96. B: In order to easily follow a client's progress, the best documentation format is a graph because it provides a visual image. Additionally, clients often like to receive feedback about their participation, and a graph can help them to note progress and encourage them to continue or to set goals for themselves. Line graphs are the most commonly used type to demonstrate improvement because they are very easy to interpret. In most cases, more than one type of documentation is used—for example, a graph may be developed with information from checklists or narratives.

97. A: If assessing a client's use of social media and the Internet in the home environment, the initial factor to assess is the client's internet access. If the client lacks access, then further assessment depends on whether the client can gain and/or afford access. Some types of access (dial up) may be less reliable than highspeed connections, and some types may be expensive. Once access is available, then the client's interest, computer knowledge, and motor skills should be assessed.

98. B: A discharge plan should include a list of barriers still present at discharge. Other important information includes diagnosis and rehabilitation problem list, goals and objectives, lists of interventions and adaptive equipment utilized, summary of progress made during the program, discharge recommendations (including leisure activities, community resources, and necessary adaptive equipment), and reasons for discharge.

99. C: The minimum period of internship necessary for the Academic Path to certification is 14 weeks/560 hours. The applicant must have received a bachelor's degree with a concentration in recreation therapy with additional support coursework. Supervision must be by a CTRS during the internship period. Two other paths are available for those seeking equivalency based on a bachelor's degree in a different field, additional coursework, and work experience in the field.

100. B: The Digit Repetition Test is used to assess attention. The individual is told to listen to numbers and then repeat them. The CTRS starts with two random single-digit numbers. If the individual gets this sequence correct, the CTRS then states three numbers and continues to add one number each time until the individual is unable to repeat the numbers correctly. People with normal intelligence (without retardation or expressive aphasia) can usually repeat 5 to 7 numbers, so scores ≤ 5 indicate impaired attention.

101. C: The professional that is most appropriate for a client who is having difficulty swallowing or communicating verbally is a speech therapist, who is able to both assess and develop a plan of treatment as well as guidelines to prevent choking and aspiration. Physical therapists evaluate and provide exercise regimens to improve or restore function. Occupational therapists evaluate abilities and assist clients to manage activities of daily living. Nurse practitioners evaluate general condition, diagnose, and treat ailments.

102. B: If the CTRS finds a client with PTSD and flashbacks cowering in the corner of the room in a state of panic, the best approach is to say, "I know you are afraid, but you are safe here." The CTRS should acknowledge the client's fears while trying to use grounding techniques to remind the client that he is safe. The CTRS should not attempt to reach out to the client or touch the client without first asking for permission as this may trigger a violent response.

103. C: Clients who are diagnosed with severe depression and engaging in recreation therapy as part of treatment should be routinely assessed for suicidal ideation because it is common with severe depression. The CTRS should ask the client directly and work with the client to develop a safety plan, such as removal of firearms from the home and creation of crisis lists of those from whom the client can seek help.

104. A: The pattern of symptoms characteristic of schizophrenic includes positive symptoms (delusions, hallucinations) or negative symptoms (flat affect, social isolation). Clients may exhibit a varying range of symptoms, depend on the severity of the disease. Poor hygiene is common. Some people hear "voices" and may respond by carrying out acts of violence, but this is rare. Depression and dual diagnosis are common co-morbidities.

105. B: Normalization refers to the conditions of a client's life being as normal as possible. That is, the client is able to live and function in the home environment, work, and socialize. Even though functioning may not be the same as before disability/injury, life can return to a new normal, and the client can live a rewarding life. The goal of normalization has fueled the movement toward deinstitutionalization and community integration for those with disabilities.

106. B: The Recreation Behavior Inventory requires the CTRS to observe a client's behavior is 20 different activities in order to evaluate skills. The CTRS observes the client for different behaviors in the cognitive (reasoning, comprehension), sensory (hearing, vision, touch), and motor (fine, gross) domains. Each item in the inventory is scored on a 3-point scale. This inventory, originally intended for use with children, is also commonly used to evaluate adults with psychiatric illness and those in long-term care.

107. A: If a recreation therapy program focuses on functional interventions to improve both physical and social functioning, the assessment that is most indicated is a functional assessment. It's important that there is a match between the program that is available to clients and the assessment in order to accurately place the client into the program so that the client receives the most benefit. For example, if the program has no components that address concentration skills, then assessing concentration will not help to place the client.

108. D: If a recreation therapy program includes many different service options, the best method of placement to ensure positive outcomes is by assessment. While client preferences should always be considered, if the client is to benefit from therapy, then the choice of services should be based on need as determined by assessment. If the program and the assessment do not match, then the client is unlikely to show progress in areas of need.

109. C: The activity that may be used to assess fine motor skills includes picking up pencils from a table top and placing in a cup. Other assessments include the box and block test in which blocks are moved from one section of a box to another section and the 9-hold peg test in which pegs are picked up, placed in a peg-board, removed, and returned to the original container. The activities are timed.

110. D: When developing an appropriate exercise plan for a client with anorexia nervosa, the CTRS should avoid discussing the relationship of calories to exercise because many clients exercise obsessively in order to lose weight and are focused on reducing calories. Often in the early stages of treatment, clients are restricted from exercise in order to break their exercise pattern. Once staged exercise begins, the fun and social aspects of exercise should be the focus. Clients may be taught to balance energy input and output.

111. C: The primary purpose of licensure is to protect the consumer by ensuring that those who represent themselves as recreation therapy specialists are appropriately qualified. However, currently only a few states require licensure for recreation therapy specialists (New Hampshire, Oklahoma, Utah, North Carolina) while California (title protection) and Washington (registration) have established other qualifications. Requirements for certification are usually driven by employers who hire only those who are certified rather than by state regulations.

112. A: The primary difference between an activity director at a long-term care facility and a CTRS is that the CTRS focuses on leisure activities as therapy in a time-limited manner with a program that is individualized for each client for whom recreation therapy is physician-ordered. The activity director, on the other hand, focuses on leisure activities as fun and generally provides general interest activities and services to all of the clients as mandated by federal regulations.

113. B: Video games may be most beneficial for a client with autism spectrum disorder who is resistive to interacting with other because many video games can be played individually, especially in the beginning. Once the client has mastered playing, the client may begin to enjoy playing with others because, while played together, the focus of video games tends to be on the game itself and interactions between avatars rather than interactions between other players, so video games are less intimidating.

114. C: Tossing and catching balls or balloons is most likely to improve gross motor skills. Other activities include jumping rope, practicing martial arts, dancing, and riding a bicycle. Activities that involve primarily the hands, such as making cards, playing Jenga, painting, and sorting beads of various sizes improve fine motor skills. Clients who have difficulty with activities of daily living (such as bathing, cooking, walking, cleaning, and transferring) benefit from exercises to improve fine and gross motor skills.

115. A: The ecological approach to therapeutic recreation addressed needed changes within the environment and considers both the needs of the individual and the environment. The environment includes not only the natural environment but the people and the community in which the client resides. The goals of therapy are to promote abilities and eliminate barriers within the environment that impede progress.

116. A: According to the attribution model of recreation therapy, the four factors that determine success or failure are:

- Ability: This is a stable internal quality.
- Effort: This is an unstable internal quality that may vary widely depending on my variables.
- Difficulty of task: This is a stable external quality.
- Luck: This is an unstable external quality that may vary but may be influenced by effort and ability.

117. B: If clients are asked who could write out the longest list of answers to simple questions in specified time periods—"How many candy bars can you name?" "How many flowers can you name?" and "How do you feel when you can't do something?"—the value of this exercise is that it encourages honest expressions of feeling. Clients get caught up in the competition and writing as quickly as possible so that they often are more honest in giving responses when a question is more serious.

118. C: The four core values of recreation therapy include:

- Right to leisure: Everyone is entitled to pursue leisure activities and to the support needed to do so.
- Autonomy: Clients have the right to make their own decisions and choices in regard to leisure activities.
- Optimal health: Clients have the right to work towards and experience optimal health and a sense of well-being.
- Quality of life: The client's assessment of life from both a subjective and objective point of view.

119. D: 4, 1, 3, 5, 2, 6. Six steps to ethical decision making (per ATRA's Ethics Committee) include:

1. Gather facts and information about the situation.
2. Assess whether an ethical problem is present.
3. Identify alternative actions.
4. Identify consequences associated with alternative actions.
5. Choose an action.
6. Evaluate the selected action.

120. D: According to the Therapeutic Recreation Outcome Model, if recreation therapy helps a client communicate better, express emotions, and value participation in recreational activities, the behavioral domains that have been addressed are social (communicate), psychological (emotions), and leisure (recreational activities). The other three behavioral domains include cognitive (learn something new), spiritual (value system, meaning), and physical (sports and other physical activities).

121. A: The four criteria for active treatment (which is treatment that is medically necessary) include (1) prescribed and supervised by a physician, (2) based on assessment and individualized treatment plan, (3) specified duration, intensity and frequency of interventions, and (4) positive outcomes expected. The client is expected to benefit from the interventions and to experience less need for ongoing medical care as a result of the interventions.

122. B: With the APIE process, APIE stands for:

- Assess: Complete assessment of the client and the client's environment.
- Plan: Includes goals and objectives as well as interventions needed to achieve these goals.
- Implement: Putting the plan into action and collecting data about results.
- Evaluate: Assessing the client's progress and attainment of expected outcomes. Modifying the plan as needed.

123. D: A type 1, outcome-oriented program is designed to a large group of clients so there is little focus on individual needs and goals. All clients receive the same program, so these programs usually are intended primarily for socialization and entertainment. Type 1 programs are most commonly used in long-term care facilities and group homes. Typical type 1 activities include watching movies or playing games, such as bingo.

124. B: Prior to taking a client or clients on an outing, such as to a community event, the CTRS should ensure the availability of a first aid kit and emergency plan. The staff members attending should be familiar with the location, including the location of bathrooms and exits. The client to staff ratio may vary depending on the clients' conditions but generally should not be more than 4:1. If the clients are traveling by motor vehicle, it should be checked for safety before use.

125. D: If a client appears intelligent and articulate and follows written directions well but repeatedly asks for oral directions to be repeated, the CTRS should suspect that the client has a hearing deficit. The CTRS should ask the client directly and determine if the client has hearing aids available or needs a referral for a hearing assessment. Speaking clearly and facing the client while speaking can help the client understand.

126. A: With reflective listening, if a client is speaking about loss and pauses, the best response is to maintain interested silence (say nothing, but look at the client, and nod the head to show interest) and to resist the urge to fill the silence with words. Especially when discussing difficult topics, clients often pause, and maintaining silence allows them time to think and explore feelings before continuing with their communication.

127. B: When assessing a mental health client for affect, if the client's affect is essentially blank and immobile, it would be classified as flat. A blunted affect is one in which emotional responses are reduced but not completely absent. An inappropriate affect is one in which the emotional response is at odds with the client's words or the situation. A bizarre affect is one that is completely disorganized.

128. B: If a client who is participating in a weight lifting program beings to overtrain, the outcome is likely to be decreased performance. Overtraining stresses the muscles and performance often declines precipitously. Undertraining can also decrease performance but less markedly and the decline is slower. Clients must be cautioned to follow protocols carefully in order to receive the most benefit.

129. A: If a client agrees to participate in activities but during the activities is sullen and makes frequent complaints, this is an example of passive-aggressive communication. Passive-aggressive clients often appear initially to be cooperative, agreeing to participate, but their underlying anger and resentment surfaces through their behavior (being sullen, complaining). Passive-aggressive communication is often an indication that the client feels powerless and is afraid to directly confront issues.

130. C: Under the IDEA requirements, a functional behavioral assessment (FBA) for children includes assessment of the following:

- Precipitating conditions: Setting, situation prior to onset of observed behavior.
- Specific behavior observed: Exact description of the behavior.
- Consequences: Events that follow the behavior (warnings, disciplinary action, attention).
- Function of the behavior: Assumed reason for the behavior (get attention, express frustration, intimidate others, express anger).

131. D: Poor penmanship may indicate a developmental disorder for a 10-year-old, but a 6-year-old is just learning to write. Indications of possible developmental delays for a 6-year-old child include peer problems (fighting, difficulty making friends or participating in play), depression, cruelty to animals, poor academic progress, speech problems, lack of fine motor skills, and inability to catch a ball or state age.

132. C: If a client does self-assessment with the CAGE tool and answers 2 of the 4 questions with "yes," this indicates a drinking problem. A "yes" answer for only one questions indicates a possible drinking problem. Questions:

C	Cutting down	Do you think about trying to cut down on drinking?
A	Annoyed at criticism	Are people starting to criticize your drinking?
G	Guilty feeling	Do you feel guilty or try to hide your drinking?
E	Eye opener	Do you increasingly need a drink earlier in the day?

133. D: The primary difference between regular tennis and wheelchair tennis is that the ball can bounce two times before being returned and only the first bounce must be within bounds. Otherwise, the rules are the same. Because of the need to move about the court quickly, specially-designed manual wheelchairs built for quick maneuvering are used instead of motorized wheelchairs. Wheelchair tennis is now part of the Paralympic Games and a number of other competitions are available.

134. C: When visiting a client in the home environment, safety is always the most important issue, so if a client is hostile, drugged, and/or intoxicated, the CTRS should reschedule the visit and leave. Other safeguards include:

- Visit during daytime hours.
- Carry a preprogrammed (police, 9-1-1, agency) cellular phone.
- Wear inexpensive clothing, jewelry, and watch.
- Carry identification (agency, organization).
- Avoid visiting high-crime areas alone.
- Report observed abuse after leaving home.
- Provide others with the schedule of visits.
- Enter a home only on invitation.

135. B: If a client with chronic alcoholism stops drinking, the first stage of withdrawal symptoms usually begins within 8 hours of cessation. Stages of alcohol withdrawal include:

- Beginning withdrawal: Usually within 8 hours with tremors, abdominal cramping, nausea and vomiting, excessive sweating, depression.
- Withdrawal: Usually within 24 hours with increased anxiety, mood swings, hypertension, rapid pulse and respirations, muscle rigidity, teeth clenching.

- Severe withdrawal: May occur within 12 hours or be delayed for 3 to 14 days with severe confusion, hallucinations, agitation and seizures. May develop delirium tremens with circulatory collapse and death.

136. D: When providing feedback to a client, the CTRS should avoid comparing the client's performance to that of others but may compare to client's previous performance, such as when focusing on improvements. Feedback should be objective and specific and may include providing suggestions for change. Negative feedback should always be given in private although constructive criticism may be given publicly. Feedback should always be given immediately when it has the most impact.

137. A: CRAFFT tool:

C	Have you ever ridden in a CAR driven by someone (including self) who was "high" or had been using alcohol or drugs?
R	Do you ever use alcohol or drugs to RELAX, feel better about yourself, or fit in?
A	Do you ever use alcohol or drugs while you are by yourself or ALONE?
F	Do you every FORGET things you did while using alcohol or drugs?
F	Do your family or FRIENDS every tell you that you should cut down on your drinking or drug use?
T	Have you ever gotten into TROUBLE while you were using alcohol or drugs?

138. B: 3, 1, 2, 4. The stages of recovery from substance abuse/addiction include:

- Initiation: Makes a commitment and enters a program or tries to control the addiction.
- Early abstinence: (First 90 days), undergoes withdrawal and is at risk for relapse because of cravings. Needs coping skills.
- Maintenance (After 90 days and up to 5 years) focuses on avoiding relapse and learning triggers. Needs to improve relationships with others and manage anger.
- Advanced recovery: (After 5 years of abstinence) must remain vigilant and may need 12-step meetings (AA, NA) or ongoing support groups or counseling.

139. A: If a client with diabetes mellitus, type 2 (non-insulin dependent) is engaging in walking and jogging, the most important focus of education is foot examination and foot care. Because walking and jogging are impact sports, the feet may easily become irritated and blistered, and diabetic clients often have impaired circulation and slow healing, so a small blister can result in an ulcer and even amputation if not attended to immediately.

140. D: If planning a program for a client and using the person-centered model of care, an essential element to include is choice. A program must be planned that meets the needs as well as the interests and preferences of the client, always respecting the client's right to self-determination in the provision of care. Person-centered care improves client satisfaction and compliance with the program because the client helped to develop it.

141. A: While all are important, when developing an individual recreation therapy program for an individual with moderate dementia in a long-term care facility, the most important factor to consider is the client's past interests and activities, which may be gleaned from the client's history or from family members or other staff members, especially if the client's confusion prevents the client from discussing interests. For example, if a client previously was engaged in work with her hands (painting, knitting, sewing), the client may enjoy coloring or folding clothes.

142. B: If the CTRS finds that there are no community-based recreational facilities that accommodate clients with disabilities, the CTRS should provide education and guidance to the facilities regarding inclusion, encouraging them to develop programs or modify existing programs. Directors of programs often are unaware of the steps they must take to facilitate inclusion and are often concerned about costs and liability, so the CTRS can provide information about these issues.

143. A: An adolescent hospitalized and under strict isolation may most benefit from playing electronic games, especially if a number of different games are available and the adolescent is able to connect with others through the Internet. In order to combat boredom and depression, the adolescent needs to be kept as busy as possible with different activities. Active activities tend to be better than passive activities, such as reading and watching TV, which require little of the adolescent in terms of engagement.

144. A: Before children and adolescents with Down syndrome engage in gymnastics or contact sports, it is most important to have the cervical spine evaluated by a physician because an abnormality at C1-C2 (atlantoaxial instability) is present in up to 30% of those with Down syndrome. These clients are at risk of spinal cord injuries with strenuous activities or those that result in twisting or pressure to this area of the spine. Physical activities are valuable to improve muscle tone, which tends to be low with Down syndrome.

145. C: A social barrier to participation in community-based recreational facilities occurs if the client does not have friends to help with transportation. Being unable to find information is a communication barrier, and being unable to afford private or public transportation is an economic barrier. If the client is reluctant to share personal information about health, this represents a privacy barrier. Clients often face multiple barriers to participation, and the CTRS and clients should anticipate these barriers and discuss ways to compensate.

146. D: If the CTRS at a long-term care facility has obtained a grant to develop an activity room, the first step should be to survey clients as to their interests, especially those most likely to take advantage of the room. An activity room may hold a wide variety of items, including gardening, music/movement, table games, floor games, video games, television and collection of movies, arts and crafts, cooking materials, and beauty supplies.

147. B: If clients are participating in a game of basketball in a gym, those with hyperactivity or attention-deficit disorders may especially become distressed because of the noise level. Sound tends to reverberate through a gym and there is usually little to damper the sound, and this can be distressing to many clients with mental or behavioral health issues, so they should be prepared in advance. In some cases, clients may benefit from earplugs.

148. C: If the CTRS has divided the gym into four areas for four different activities (throwing hoops, badminton, gymnastics, and weight lifting) that are going on at the same time, this practice increases the risk of injury and is a safety concern. Only one activity at a time should take place in a gym, and each activity should be adequately supervised because one person cannot safely supervise 4 different activities even if only one client is involved in each activity.

149. A: The response that is an example of therapeutic communication with a client who states that an activity is too difficult is, "Let's talk about how we can make this activity easier for you." This response engages the client in problem-solving while acknowledging the client's concerns. It's important not to compare the client with others or to focus on the negative aspects. Telling a client to "hang in there" suggests that the client has no cause for concern and ignores the client's feelings.

150. C: If a client consistently scores 4 in ability to perform tasks on the Functional Independence Measure (FIM), the percentage of the required effort for the task the client is able to achieve is 75%. Functionality level:

1. Total assistance, can use less than 25% of necessary effort for tasks.
2. Maximum assistance, can use less than 50% of necessary effort.
3. Moderate assistance, can use 50% of necessary effort.
4. Minimum assistance, can use 75% of necessary effort.
5. Supervision and minimal assistance needed.
6. Modified independence with slight help.
7. Completely independent, no assistance.

It's Your Moment, Let's Celebrate It!

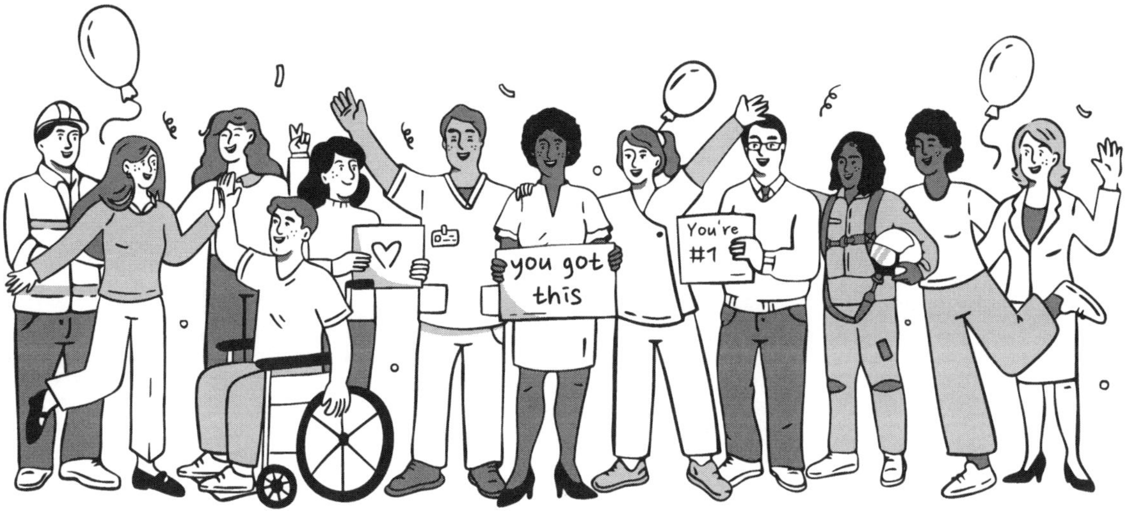

Share your story @mometrixtestpreparation